IMPORTANT NOTICE

WHAT IS AN ERRATA SHEET?

An erratum or corrigendum (plurals: errata, corrigenda) is a correction of a book. Errata are most commonly issued after the original text was published. As a general rule, publishers issue an erratum for a production error (i.e. an error introduced during the publishing process) and a corrigendum for a typesetter error.

ERRATA (Latin word for corrections)

During the editing process of this publication the wrong file was sent to the printers for this edition. We have listed the corrections so you will not think that any of the questions are missing and why some are repeated.

On page 59 the question begins with 729. and ends with 743. and on page 60 the questions begin with 772. and ends with 787.

On page 61 the questions continue in the proper sequence. The typesetter typed the wrong question numbers on those pages but there are no missing questions in the book. Just the question numbers were incorrect due to 'copying and pasting', etc.

You will find that there are several questions repeated throughout this edition and are worded slightly differently as they appear different on the exams at times. This was done purposely as those particular questions are frequently given on massage exams each year.

Section V begins with single spacing. We did this in order to include questions from our very first edition Massage Exam Study Guide in 1990 as many schools used this book in their class room setting. That section was inserted so students would have additional information for preparing to take any massage exam. Section VI continues with double spacing.

The author of this book is a Retired AMTA (American Massage Therapy Association) instructor and over the years she has found that students retain answers to questions when there is just one answer vs. multiple choices. Multiple choices tend to confuse students and a study guide is to help the students retain the answers.

We invite you to visit our web site and

www.massagenationalexam.con

D1550865

CLICK ON ENDORSEMENTS link and you will see why our massage study guides have been, and still are, the best-selling books each year since 1990. See what present and past students have to say about our books on the endorsement page. We have also included what students are saying about our new 2009 Edition on Amazon. It is our desire that you have as many questions as possible that are given on all exams. Thank you for ordering the book.

Publisher

Massage National Exam State & Canadian Exams Study Guide

Daphna R. Moore
Retired AMTA Massage Instructor

Hughes Henshaw Publications, LLC
Palm Bay, FL

Massage National Exam
State & Canadian Exams Study Guide
2009 Edition

Published by Hughes Henshaw Publications LLC
1871 Red Bud Circle NW
Palm Bay, FL 32907
321-956-8885 • Fax: 321-956-2475
www.massagenationalexam.com
email: hugheshenshaw@aol.com

Moore, Daphna
    Massage National Exam, State & Canadian Exams Study Guide – First Edition

ISBN 978-1-892693-39-6

1. Massage Therapy 2. Massage Exams 3. Massage Therapy Study Guides

We thank the following individuals: Cherie Sohnen-Moe, with Sohnem-Moe Associated, Inc., **www.sohnen-moe.com** for granting permission to use the forms and charts in this publication, pages 111-114. There were taken from her book "Business Mastery," ISBN 0-9621265-4-4 and we highly recommend her book titled, "The Ethics of Touch" co-authored with Ben E. Benjamin, Ph.D., ISBN 1-882908-40-6.

We thank James D. Smith, LMT with Healing With Massage at **www.Smithmethod.com** for permission to use quotes on pages 109-110. Mr. Smith's practice has been nominated "Best of Long Island" by the Long Island Press. You can reach Mr. Smith at (631-724-7621).

Hughes Henshaw Publications LLC

Palm Bay, FL 32907

About The Author

In 1976 I attended Lotus Lodge, a Wholistic Retreat in Strasburg, OH, taking various modalities: massage, iridology, nutrition, color therapy, etc. In the summer of 1979 and 1980 I attended classes at the Healing Light Center in Glendale, CA with Roslyn Bruyer and studied Aura Balancing, energy modalities, etc. In 1980 and 1981 I took a 6-month class on Touch for Health© Textbook by John F. Thie, D.C. in Boulder, CO. This included muscle testing, meridians and oriental philosophy. I became a member of the AMTA in February 1986, (graduated under a previous married name) and have continued my studies and create various tests for students in order to help them pass massage certification exams.

In 1989 and 1990 I attended a few workshops at the Colorado School of Traditional Chinese Medicine in Denver, CO. These classes were for gaining knowledge and not for any credit toward a degree. I also studied ANMA, the art of Japanese Massage, In Boulder, CO, not for credit but for additional knowledge. During 1980 I took classes in hypnosis in Denver, CO, and became a hypno-therapist in 1981 utilizing this for past life regressions.

My purpose in publishing this book is to help students prepare for any exam, whether they are exams they are having in school, final exams, or for any Massage Certification, i.e. school exams, state board exams, MBLEx and National exams. The questions in this book are not broken down into categories. Over the years I have found that students retain the answers if there are not too many choices to choose from. The books listed below are just some of the many books I have studied throughout the years and have created questions from these books as well as articles that have been in various massage magazines since 1989. I continue to network with many instructors throughout the country and am still a 'student-at-heart' as massage and healing modalities are constantly finding new ways and techniques for healing the body, mind and spirit.

Healing Massage Techniques, Holistic, Classic, & Emerging Methods Second Edition, Frances M. Tappen© 1980
Touch For Health© 1979, textbook by John F. Thie, D.C.
Pain Erasure,© Bonnie Pruden 1980
Structure & Function of the Body© 1992, Mosby
Stedman's Concise Medical Dictionary© 1987
Essential Pathology © Emanuel Rubin, 1989
The Foundations of Chinese Medicine© Giovanni Maciocia 1989
The Practice of Chinese Medicine© 1989 Giovanni Maciocia
Human Anatomy and Physiology© Elaine Marieb 1989
Mosby's Fundamentals of Therapeutic Massage© Sandy Fritz 2004
A Massage Therapist's Guide to Pathology© Ruth Werner 1998
Milady's Theory and Practice of Therapeutic Massage© 1999 Mark F. Beck
Trail Guide to the Body© 1997 Andrew Biel
The Ethics of Touch© 2003 Ben E. Benjamin, Ph.D., and Cherie Sohnen-Moe
Business Mastery © 1988 Cherie M. Sohnen-Moe
The Eastern Bodyworker's StudyGuide© 1999 Derek Brigham
Taber's Cyclopedic Medical Dictionary© 1963 Clarence Wilbur Taber
The Original Reiki Handbook of Dr. Mikao Usui© 1998 Dr. Kikao Usui and Frank Arjava Petter
Stedman's Concise Medical Dictinary © 1987 Williams & Wilkins
Anma, The Art of Japanese Massage© 1995 Mochizuki
Clinical Massage Therapy© 2000 Fiona Rattray and Linda Ludwig

TRUE & FALSE and FILL IN THE BLANKS
QUESTIONS & ANSWERS
SECTION I

1.   *TRUE OR FALSE.* Thai massage uses pressure on the meridian lines to open sens, (another name for energy lines in the body.) **TRUE. Thai uses pressure.**

2.   *TRUE OR FALSE.* Shiatsu massage incorporates using the fingers, thumbs, and palm with pressure along the meridians. **TRUE**

3.   *TRUE OR FALSE.* Trigger Point massage applies finger pressure to the areas in the muscles that are tender in order to help stop pain and any muscle spasms. **TRUE**

4.   *TRUE OR FALSE.* Acupuncture uses hot stones to correct energy imbalances in the body. **FALSE. Acupuncture uses and inserts very delicate needles into the skin at various points along the channel or meridians to correct energy imbalances.**

5.   *TRUE OR FALSE.* Acupressure is very similar to Shiatsu because it, too, uses finger point massage pressure to help release tension in the muscles. **TRUE**

6.   *TRUE OR FALSE.* The deep heat of the stones in Warm/Hot Stone Therapy provides a quick relaxation response. **TRUE**

7.   *TRUE OR FALSE.* Reiki is a system of energy healing that comes from Japan. In Reiki, the therapist places both of their hands very gently in certain positions on the body and/or above the body. This is referred to as *laying-on-of-hands* and it is designed to relieve pain, to heal physical illnesses, and help the spiritual growth. The therapist transmits the life energy (Qi, Ki, or Chi) to the electro-magnetic energy field around the body to help healing processes. **TRUE**

8.   *TRUE OR FALSE.* Swedish massage uses very fine needles on certain parts of the body. **FALSE. Swedish massage uses five basic massage strokes which are effleurage, tapotement, friction, vibration, and petrissage.**

9.   *TRUE OR FALSE.* Effleurage uses gliding strokes. **TRUE**

10.   *TRUE OR FALSE.* Tapotement uses percussion tapping and pounding. **TRUE**

11.   *True of False.* Petrissage uses kneading and compression strokes. **TRUE**

12.   *TRUE OR FALSE.* Friction uses a deep circular rubbing. **TRUE**

13.   *TRUE OR FALSE.* Vibration uses a very fine movement and also rapid shaking. **TRUE**

14. *TRUE OR FALSE.* Ayurvedic's originated from India and this type of massage can include using special oils, massaging the scalp and body kneading. Two therapists are used many times in this modality and ayurvedic massage helps to remove and unblock the energy flow so the body can begin healing itself. **TRUE**

15. *TRUE OR FALSE.* Sports and Athletic Massage incorporates stretching and compression techniques, promotes fast recovery from injuries, reduces the blood pressure and heart rate, relieves muscle tension and chronic muscle pain, restores ROM (range of motion) and improves flexibility. It also enhances the athletic performance and it can be used before and after competitions. **TRUE**

16. *TRUE OR FALSE.* Acute inflammation or injury is very common among sporting events. It is only after the swelling and pain begin to subside that you can begin to apply sports massage. The time element for the acute stage of an injury, to where you cannot massage, is the first 72 hours after an injury. **TRUE**

17. *TRUE OR FALSE.* Reflexology is an ancient Chinese application. It not only utilizes pressure points on the feet, but also on the ears and hands, that match up to certain areas of the body. **TRUE**

18. *TRUE OR FALSE.* Tui Na is now being used by many therapists in the USA and it focuses more on certain problems instead of an overall general massage session. It is an excellent adjunct to Swedish Massage as its major focus of application utilizes acupressure points, the energy channels (meridians), specific pain areas, muscles, and joints. Also this technique incorporates the utilization of compresses, poultices and some salves. **TRUE**

19. *TRUE OR FALSE.* Aromatherapy incorporates the use of essential oils that are applied to the body. Everyone can benefit from massages using essential oils. **TRUE**

20. *TRUE OR FALSE.* In Oriental Medicine the examinations are usually done at the initial interview. **TRUE**

21. *TRUE OR FALSE.* When you have a client that has scheduled several appointments with you, and you, for *whatever reason*, become uncomfortable with that client and no longer want to work with the client. You should tell the client you are uncomfortable with them and no longer want to have them as a client. **FALSE. You should just refer the person to another therapist.**

22. *TRUE OR FALSE.* METs are one of the most valuable tools that a massage therapist can have in the 'tool box.' **TRUE**

23. *TRUE OR FALSE.* The 3 parts of the Assessment are taking the client's history, observation, and taking their temperature. **FALSE. The 3 parts are taking the history, observation and examination.**

24.   *TRUE OR FALSE.* Palpation is a primary form of assessment and when palpating soft tissue it can help the therapist determine the client's normal soft tissue detect lesions or pathology in the tissue. **TRUE**

25.   *TRUE OR FALSE.* In Oriental Medicine, at your first initial examination there are two ways to examine - looking at the tongue and taking your pulse. **TRUE**

26.   *TRUE OR FALSE.* You stop artificial respiration when the person resumes breathing. **TRUE**

27.   *TRUE OR FALSE.* In giving CPR the head-tilt, chin-lift maneuver would prevent the tongue from blocking the airway passage. **TRUE**

28.   *TRUE OR FALSE.*   Deoxygenated blood is returned from the body into the right atrium. **TRUE**

29.   *TRUE OR FALSE.* Force on a joint many cause it to pop-out of its socket and this would be called a dislocation. **TRUE**

30.   *TRUE OR FALSE.* If you find yourself in a position where you must do CPR, the best position for the person to be in when you are doing CPR is for them to be flat on the floor. **TRUE**

31.   *TRUE OR FALSE.*   After you call 911 to report a cardiac arrest, you should start CPR immediately. It may save a life. **TRUE**

32.   *TRUE OR FALSE.* The ratio of chest compressions to ventilation in an adult person is 30 to 2. **TRUE**

33.   *TRUE OR FALSE.* If a person has had bypass surgery and something happens that they require CPR, you should do CPR in the regular manner. **TRUE**

34.   *TRUE OR FALSE.* You can get sued if you perform CPR? **TRUE but there has never been a successful suit brought against someone performing CPR.**

35.   *TRUE OR FALSE.* If you are alone and you don't know CPR you should call 911 and ask the emergency dispatcher to give you instructions over the phone. **TRUE**

36.   *TRUE OR FALSE.* The cervical vertebrae are different from all the other vertebrae (thoracic, lumbar, sacral, and coccygeal) because they possess transverse foramina in order for the vertebral arteries to pass through on their way to the foramen magnum, (which is one of the several circular apertures in the base of the skull through which the medulla oblongata enters and exits the skull.) **TRUE**

37.   *TRUE OR FALSE.* The term 'triage' refers to low back pain and the 3(triage) groupings being: serious spinal pathology, nerve root pain, and non-specific causes. **TRUE**

38.   *TRUE OR FALSE.* Impostor symptoms are symptoms that imitate as back pain. **TRUE**

39.   *TRUE OR FALSE.* You have a client who is lying in a supine position (lying flat) and you ask the client to medially rotate (which means rotate toward the center of the body) and flex the knee, the muscle that would be used to do this would be the popliteus.   **TRUE**

40.   You must study about isotonic, isometric, eccentric and concentric.

Most massage schools throughout the country will have questions on these four things and will give situations where you will have to tell whether something is isotonic, isometric, eccentric or concentric. When I was an AMTA Massage Instructor years ago, I would put this on my exams. **About MET (Muscle Energy Techniques).** MET are a class of soft tissue manipulation methods that incorporate precisely directed and controlled patient initiated, isometric and/or isotonic contractions designed to improve musculoskeletal function & reduce pain.

Isometric contraction is one in which a muscle, or group of muscles, or a joint, or region of the body, is called upon to contract or move in a specific direction, and in which that effort is matched by the practitioner/therapist's effort, so that no movement is allowed to take place.

Isotonic contractions in which movement does take place, in that the counterforce offered by the therapist is either less than that of the patient, or is greater. In the first isotonic example there would be an approximation of the origin and insertion of the muscle(s) involved, as the effort exerted by the patient more than matches that of the therapist. This has a tonic effect on the muscle(s) and is called a concentric isotonic contraction. This method is useful in toning weakened musculature.

The other form of isotonic contraction involves an eccentric movement in which the muscle, while contracting, is stretched. The effect of the therapist offering greater counterforce than the patient's muscular effort is to lengthen a muscle which is trying to shorten. This is called an isolytic contraction when performed rapidly. This maneuver is useful in cases where there exists a marked degree of fibrotic change. The effect is to stretch and alter these tissues – inducing controlled microtrauma – thus allowing an improvement in elasticity and circulation. When the eccentric isotonic stretch is performed slowly, the effect is to tone the muscle being stretched, while simultaneously inhibiting the antagonists, which can subsequently be stretched.[1] We would like to thank Dr. Leon Chaitow, Honorary Fellow, University of Westminster, London for giving us permission to reprint the above number 40. From his book *Muscle Energy Techniques*.

41. What kind of insurance should a therapist obtain for their protection against an accident and/or malpractice? **Liability Insurance**

42. *TRUE OR FALSE.* Massage therapists do not have to keep accurate records as long as their clients schedule appointments regularly. **FALSE.**

43. *TRUE OR FALSE.* The method used which fixes the calcaneus (the subtalar joint) and circumducts the forefoot is the circumduction test. **TRUE.**

44. *TRUE OR FALSE.* The client's Intake Form is essential for the first visit in order to obtain their personal health and history information. **TRUE**

45. *TRUE OR FALSE.* The epididymis is part of the male reproductive system? **TRUE. It is a structure within the scrotum near the testes.**

46. *TRUE OR FALSE.* In Ayurvedic the three doshas are Vata, Pitta, and QiGong. **FALSE, they are Kapha, Pitta and Vata.**

47. *TRUE OR FALSE.* In Ayurvedic, Pitta is referred to as fire. **TRUE**

48. *TRUE OR FALSE.* In Arurvedic, Vata types are creative, Kapha types are patient and usually solidly built, and Pitta types are firey and they tend to be impatient and they should avoid spicy foods. **TRUE**

49. *TRUE OR FALSE.* In Arurvedic there is something called time elements. There are time periods throughout each day that describes how our energy levels are functioning. From 2 am to 6 am and 2 pm to 6 pm is referred to as Vata times and during this time you will have a lot of creativity but your physical energy tends to be low, and from 6 am to 10 am and from 6 pm to 10pm, it is referred to at the Kapha times and during this time you tend to be lethargic. From 10 am to 2 pm and from 10 pm to 2 am it is referred to as Pitta times and referred to as firey energy. **TRUE**

50. **This is not a question. It is for you to study thoroughly.**

In The Chinese Time Clock theory, the time clock is universal. There are two reasons/causes of disease according to the Chinese. They are lack of blood flow to the various organ/s, and lack of energy to the organ. Our energy starts circulating in the body from 3-5am. According to the Chinese we only need approximately 3-4 hours of sleep IF our body is in perfect balance.

The time element for the organs are as follows:

Note: When I was in school in the late 1980s, we were given questions on the energy meridians and channels. Our questions ranged from "What time would the energy for the liver meridian be most active?" Of course, it would be 1-3 am. Remember the times, the meridians, and the organs, as questions can be stated in many different styles. I always preferred no multiple choice questions on the tests I would create for students as it helped to eliminate any confusion for the 'test-takers.'

Study the below thoroughly. When I list Lung it also means lung meridian, stomach also means stomach meridian, etc. I will have charts in the back of this book.

3-5 am Lung and the Lung meridian is paired with the large intestine; **5-7 am** Large Intestine; **7-9 am** Stomach and the stomach meridian is paired with the spleen and pancreas;

9-11 am Spleen – Pancreas. Note: The spleen is part of the immune system and the spleen makes our blood and is involved in both the red and white cell formation. The Pancreas produces red blood cells; **11 am – 1 pm** Heart, and the heart meridian is paired with the small intestine; **1-3 pm** Small Intestine (where most of the digestion takes place); **5-7 pm** Kidney (Adrenal Glands); **7-9 pm** Heart Constrictor; **9-11 pm** Triple Heater which controls digestion, excretion, respiration. (Is referred to as the body's temperature and energy zone); The Triple heater does not have a corresponding organ but certainly has a meridian as the organs involved in this are the thyroid, adrenal/kidney and the lungs. Sometimes it is called the body's furnace. **1-3 am** Liver, and the liver meridian is paired with the gall bladder and the liver stores glycogen as well as distributes sustenance.

51. *TRUE OR FALSE.* In the five element theory, the elements are fire, metal, water, earth, and wood and in the design of a five pointed start, it includes the emotions/traits, climates, seasons, taste, and the five elements are constantly interacting with each other in order to bring about changes and the Qi or Chi (energy) circulates throughout the organs every 24 hours. **TRUE**

52. **This is not a question**.

In the five element theory the elements are as follows:

Wood relates to the **liver**, the trait is **anger** and the taste is **sour**
Fire relates to the **heart** and **sexual glands**, the trait is **arrogance** and **impatience** and the taste is **bitter.**
Earth relates to the **stomach**, the trait is **worry** and the taste is **sweet.**
Metal relates to the **lungs**, the trait is **sadness**, and the taste is **spicy.**
Water relates to the **kidneys**, the taste is **salty** and the trait is **fear.**

53. *TRUE OR FALSE.* The Governing vessel originates from the perineum just before the anus, runs in the midline up along the spinal column and reaches the head. This meridian meets all the Yang meridians. In

TCM is it referred to as the **sea of the yang meridians.** It is responsible for governing the energy (Qi) for all the yang meridians of the body. **TRUE**

54.   *TRUE OR FALSE.* The Conception vessel originates from the perineum, runs along the anterior midline of the abdomen, passes through the cheek and enters into the eye socket finally. It runs along the front of the body and it meets all the yin meridians, and thus is called the **sea of the yin meridians.** It is responsible for receiving and bearing the energy (Qi) of the yin meridians. In women, this meridian is thought to originate in the uterus. **TRUE**

55.   *TRUE OR FALSE.* The Girdling Vessel originates below the rib side and it runs in a downward path along the lateral side of the loin and encircles the waist. It passes through the uterus like a girdle, and it retains the meridians of the entire body. **TRUE**

56.   *TRUE OR FALSE.* It would be okay to use hydrotherapy if your patient has the following: diabetes, very high blood pressure, or any infections. **FALSE**

57.   *TRUE OR FALSE.* Applying cold packs or ice would help to reduce inflammation, muscle spasms, and reduce swelling. **TRUE**

58.   How many main charkas are there? **Seven**

59.   What is Anatomy? **A study of the structure of the   body.**

60.   What is Physiology? **A study of the functions of the body.**

61.   Name and locate the vital force which controls all body functions. **The brain is the vital force that controls all body functions.**

62.   Name the upper and lower extremities. **Upper: shoulders, arms, forearms, and hands Lower: Thighs, legs, and feet**

63.   Cartilage is from what kind of tissue? **Connective tissue**

64.   Name the three fundamental movements of Swedish massage. **Effleurage, Tapotement, and Petrissage**

65.   What movement is always used in general body massage? **Effleurage**

66.   Briefly discuss the therapeutic effects of Effleurage. **Helps in cases of fatigue and insomnia, reduces swelling and congestion, helps in cases of sprains, and power to stimulate circulation.**

67.   What type of massage is especially useful in insomnia? **Effleurage**

68.   List the things where effleurage can be used and/or is beneficial. **(1) treat someone with digestive problems, (2) used in transition from one stoke to another, (3) deep manipulation of soft tissue, (4) to break up areas of fibrosis, use deep effleurage, (5) treating tennis elbow by deep stroking and soothing effleurage,**

(6) to promote lymphatic flow, (7) to begin massage session, (8) relieving tension in the tibialis anterior,(9)   effleurage is used before petrissage movement, and (10) effleurage is one of the four basic movements in massage, (11) has a calming effect on the nervous system, (12) relieves recurrent shoulder dislocation after surgery, (13) used first in massaging the lower extremities, (14) adequate to perform fascia adherons, (15) one of the six manipulations used in Swedish massage.

69.   Should massage ever the cause client discomfort? **NO**

70.   Name the four general classifications of bones and give one example of each. **Long=Femur   Short=Patella   Irregular=Vertebrae Flat=Scapula**

71.   Name at least three important functions of the skeleton. **(1) protection of organs, (2) acts as framework for the body's means of locomotion, and (3) source of attachment of muscles.**

72.   How many named bones are found in the adult skeleton? **206**

73.   What is periosteum and what are the functions of periosteum? **Periosteum is the fibrous membrane that covers practically all bones in the body, acting both as a means of blood supply for the bones and an attachment for many of the muscles of the body.**

74.   What vital force activates all muscle function? **Nerves**

75.   Briefly describe Petrissage manipulation. **Use a kneading motion by grasping your client's skin with your hands and intermittent compression against the underlying bony surface. The purpose is for stimulating underlying tissue and muscle. Pressure should always be applied in an upward direction and always in line with the bone. You don't twist the muscles.**

76.   How does Petrissage differ form Effleurage? **With effleurage you use your entire hand or both hands and you stroke the body in only one direction; the deeper stroking is normally with the venous flow, while the light stroking can be against the venous flow. Effleurage induces relaxation. You also use the tips of your fingers while doing effleurage and keep your hands and fingers relaxed, not rigid. Petrissage is a deeper, kneading, circular motion.**

77.   Which of the above, petrissage or effleurage is most stimulating to the tissues? **Petrissage**

78.   Why is petrissage valuable in the after treatment of fractures? **It draws additional nutrition to the area primarily and gives the maximum effect in emptying and refilling the blood vessels and lymph spaces and channels.**

79.   Name the three types of muscle found in the body.

Voluntary muscles (Straited or cross striped) are skeletal muscles and are found attached to bones.
Involuntary muscles (non-straited or smooth) are found in the walls of blood vessels in the alimentary, genital and urinary systems, and control the movements of the stomach and intestines.
Cardiac muscles are intermediate in character between voluntary and involuntary. The cardiac muscles are associated with the pumping action of the heart.

80.   What type of muscle controls the size of the pupil of the eye? **Involuntary**

81.   What is muscle tone? **When muscle fibers are constantly in a state of slight contraction.**

82.   Do the muscles of an athlete contain more muscle fibers than the person who does not exercise? **No. The muscle just increases in size.**

83.   In Chinese medicine, what is used for effective digestion? **Ginseng and ginko**

84.   What is homeostasis? **A state of balance where all body systems are working in an appropriate manner.**

85.   In sagittal plane, the ulna is distal to what? **Wrist**

86.   *TRUE OR FALSE.* The extension is not effective because of the muscles that surround the area. **TRUE**

87.   *TRUE OR FALSE.* Cellulose can be digested by humans. **FALSE**

88.   Which chakra is related to the heart? **Fourth**

89.   What color chakra is related to the heart? **Green; however, some books refer to it as pink.**

90.   *TRUE OR FALSE.* The inner ear is related to the gallbladder meridian. **TRUE**

91.   *TRUE OR FALSE.* In Chinese medicine the main physiological processes in the middle burner does not relate to digestion. **FALSE. It does relate to digestion.**

92.   Which tissue helps to connect muscle to bone? **Tendon**

93.   What do ligaments do for the body? **Movement of the joints**

94.   Your client would _____ for a gait test. **Walk**

95.   How would you know about your client's past injuries or medical problems? During the interview you would get their medical history.

96. Can the application of heat help your client? If it can, how would it help them and what would be one type of therapy that would be used? **Warm hydrotherapy is one method and by applying warmth it helps your client to feel more comfortable and in many cases it can bring about the release of endorphins which makes the body feel good and can in many cases release pain.**

97. *TRUE OR FALSE.* According to the Department of Health, if an elderly woman around 65-75 years of age who has a history of drinking and smoking and is especially small-boned, she might be more likely to develop osteoporosis. **TRUE**

98. What could cause sympathetic dystrophy disease? **Several things can cause this i.e. any irritation and abnormal excitation of nervous tissue that could happen after surgery, arthritis can cause this as well.**

99. Yes or No. If you have a client who seems to be in denial about their pain and frustrations and can't seem to give you correct feedback about their situation/s, would this be referred to as a coping strategy? **YES**

100. If you had a client who had an injury of the foot and it appears it did not heal normally and looks red and is hot to the touch, what could they possibly have? **Sympathetic dystrophy disease.**

101. What causes lordosis? **Poor posture, weak quadrate lumborum, neuromuscular problems, back surgery, etc.**

102. How can a therapist help their client with scoliosis? **By applying St. John Neoromuscular Therapy because it has good results treating idiopathic and postural scoliosis.**

103. What should you do if your client has a seizure attack on the table during a treatment? **Hold the client on the table so they will not fall off.**

104. What part of the body does lordosis affect? **Lower lumbar**

105. Would poor circulation of the blood flow affect the healing of cartilage? **YES**

106. Can massage therapy help someone with Rheumatoid arthritis, and how? **Yes. It would help to circulate the synovial fluids.**

107. What is Torticollis? **Wryneck**

108. What are other names for Wryneck? **Sore neck, twisted neck, stiff neck, and spasmodic torticollis.**

109. How is lordosis described in the body? **Curvature of the spine**

110. What are the first symptoms of osteoarthritis? **Swelling and heat.**

111. What is goiter and where is it located? **It is an enlargement of the thyroid gland located just below the Adam's Apple.**

112. Are coughing and wheezing associated with Asthma and bronchitis? **YES**

113. *TRUE OR FALSE.* Anemia is caused by Vitamin B12 deficiency. **TRUE**

114. What nutrient helps with the formation of our bones and our teeth? **Vitamin D—It promotes absorption of calcium and magnesium, which are essential for the normal development of healthy teeth and bones.**

115. What should a therapist due if a client shows up under the influence of alcohol? **Tell the client that they will have to reschedule.**

116. What does myocardial infarction refer to? **Heart attack**

117. *TRUE OR FALSE.* The glenohumeral joint consists of the humerus and scapula. **TRUE**

118. *TRUE OR FALSE.* The glenohumerl joint is a gliding joint. **FALSE. It is a ball and socket joint.**

119. What skin infection is contagious from person to person contact? **Impetigo**

120. Which muscle (thick muscle) is hard to palpitate in the triangle of the neck? **Sternocleidomastoid muscle**

121. *TRUE OR FALSE.* Massaging the sternocleidomastoid muscle can help relieve vertigo? **TRUE**

122. *TRUE OR FALSE.* The urogentital system includes sex organs, urinary system, and the excretion of the vertebrates. **TRUE**

123. *TRUE OR FALSE.* Integument is the enveloping membrane of the body. **TRUE**

124. Which does the integument include? **Dermis and epidermis**

125. *TRUE OR FALSE.* Hydrotherapy cannot have an effect on the superficial integument. **FALSE. It can have an effect.**

126. What causes tendonitis? **Overuse of the muscle.**

127. What two organs are related to the earth element in oriental medicine? **Spleen and Pancreas**

128. Where does the stomach meridian begin and end? **Begins below the center of the eye, it descends down the center of the throat, through the chest, nipples, abdomen and groin where it jogs**

over and down the outside of the center of the leg, over the instep, ending at the base of the second toe.

129. Where does the large intestine meridian begin and end? **Begins on the index finger and travels along the arm, over the shoulder to the end on the face just to the outside of the nose.**

130. What is another name for meridian? **Pathway**

131. Where does the spleen meridian begin and end? **Begins on the big toe, travels along the arch of the foot and continues up the inside of the leg to the torso.**

132. Where does the heart meridian begin and end? **Begins in the armpit, travels along the inside of the arm and ends on the little finger.**

133. Where does the small intestine meridian begin and end? **Begins on the outside tip of the pinky finger, runs along the back of the arm, across the shoulder blade and onto the face, ending in front of the ear.**

134. When promoting reflexology, the therapist can identify a problem because of what? **Tightness in certain areas of the feet, sand like substances, and extreme tender areas of the feet.**

135. What type of movement is related with moving the body from its longitudinal? **Extension**

136. What type of modality penetrates deep tissue muscle? **Shaitsu**

137. What two contraindications would you have in Trager? **Blood clots and massaging on joints that have had surgery less than three (3) months.**

138. Which hormone is related to the sympathetic system? **Cortisol Insulin-Oxytocin**

139. Yes or No. Is it contraindicated to do heavy percussion below the thoracic region? **YES**

140. What is the largest organ? **The skin**

141. What muscle relaxes when inhalation is involved? **Diaphragm**

142. What organ is affected in a long term disease? **Liver**

143. Which tubes are responsible to conduct urine from the kidneys to the urinary bladders? **Ureters**

144. When is Active free range of motion performed. **It is performed when the client actively contracts the muscles crossing a joint, moving the joint through the unrestricted range.**

145. The muscle contracts and shortens against a constant load would be_____. **Isotonic**

146. What two muscles are antagonistic to each other? **Biceps and triceps.**

147. What is the correct way to lift an object? **Bend from your knees so you are close to the object and do not rotate your stance and face the object you are lifting and do not bend from the waist.**

148. *TRUE OR FALSE.* Physiologic effects of massage are beneficial. **TRUE**

149. What type of movement should be applied to shoulder pain? **First you would do Range of Motion (ROM) if pain is not to severe and then palpation around the area.**

150. *TRUE OR FALSE.* The purpose of stretching is to improve mobility and flexibility. **TRUE**

151. By providing first aid, how many breaths per minute does an adult need? **2 breaths for every 30 compressions**

152. *TRUE OR FALSE.* RICE (rest, ice, compression, elevation) is used for a soft tissue injury. **TRUE**

153. In Chinese medicine, acupressure is fulfilled/corrected when the body_____. **Is in balance**

154. Give three reasons why yoga is effective. **(1) the exercises emotionally and mentally help to control the bodily functions (2) helps relieve stress, and (3) helps decrease your blood pressure.**

155. What are moral principles? **The difference between right and wrong, maintaining a code of ethics and respecting people's boundaries. Be sure and know the Code of Ethics of Bodywork and Massage practices and principles. Excellent book to study would be Cherie M. Sohnen-Moe's books.**

156. In a dual-role relationship, the massage therapist is violating the code of ethics when they_____. **Ask their client out socially, i.e. a date or can I call you sometime to chat.**

157. **TRUE OR FALSE.** In business, what remains after subtracting all the cost i.e. depreciation, interest, taxes, from their company's revenues is called the net profit income. **TRUE**

158. *TRUE OR FALSE.* An individual's net income is used to determine how much income tax is owed. **TRUE**

159. What structural unit forms all the material in the body? **Cells**

ORIGINS, INSERTIONS, AND ACTIONS OF MUSCLES
QUESTIONS 1-100 that follows

1.   What is the insertion of the zygomaticus? **Zygomatic bone**

2.   What is the insertion of the adductor magnus? **Linea aspera of femur, and adductor tubercle of femur**

3.   What is the insertion of the levator scapula? **Superior angle of scapula**

4.   What is the insertion of the tibialis anterior? **First cuneiform and the first metatarsal**

5.   What is the origin of the temporalis? **Temporal bone**

6.   What is the insertion of the trapezius? **Base of spine scapula, clavicle, and acromion**

7.   What is the insertion of the spinalis thoracis? **Spines of middle and upper thoracic vertebrae**

8.   What is the insertion of the vastus medialis? **Common tendon of quadriceps femoris, also referred to as tibial tuberosity, and patella**

9.   What is the action of the vastus medialis? **Extends leg and draws patella inward**

10. What is the insertion of the adductor brevis? **Upper third of medial lip of linea aspera of femur (pubis)**

11. What is the insertion of the tensor fascia late? **Iliotibial band of fascia lata**

12. What is the insertion of the extensor digitorum brevis? **To 1st phalanx of great toe and the tendons of extensor digitorum longus, of 4 medial toes (not 5th toe)**

13. What is the insertion of the semimembranosus? **Posterior medial condyle of the tibia**

14. What is the insertion of the pectineus? **Pectineal line of femur**

15. What is the insertion of the soleus? **Calcaneus, by way of the Achilles tendon**

16. What is the insertion of the depressor anguli oris? **Angle of mouth**

17. What is the insertion of the buccinator? **Orbicularis oris**

18. What is the insertion of the brachialis? **Ulnar tuberosity, coronoid process**

19.   What is the insertion of teres minor? **Inferior facet on greater tubercle of humerus**

20.   What is the origin of the teres minor? **Axillary border of scapula**

21.   What is the action of the teres minor? **Rotates arm outward, and extension of humerus**

22.   What is the action of the teres major? **Rotates arm inward, draws it down in the back**

23.   What is the insertion of the teres major? **Medial lip of the bicipital groove of the humerus**

24.   What is the origin of the teres major? **Inferior angle of the scapula**

25.   What is the action of the pectoralis major? **Flexes, adducts and rotates arm**

26.   What is the origin of the pectoralis major? **Sternum, clavicle and cartilages of 1st through 6th ribs**

27.   What is the insertion of the pectoralis major? **Bicipital groove of humerus**

28.   What is the insertion of the pectoralis minor? **Coracoid process of scapula**

29.   What is the insertion of the supraspinatus? **Greater tubercle of the humerus**

30.   What is the action of the infraspinatus? **Extension of humerus and lateral rotation**

31.   What is the insertion of the coracobrachialias? **Middle of inner border of humerus**

32.   What is the origin of the coracobrachialias? **Coracoid process of scapula (flexion of shoulder)**

33.   What is the insertion of the brachioradialis? **Styloid process of the radius**

34.   What is the origin of the brachioradialis? **Brachioradialis originates from the proximal 2/3 of the lateral supracondylar ridge of the humerus, and the anterior surface of the lateral intermuscular septum supracondylar ridge of humerus; sometimes called the shaft of the humerus**

35.   What is the action of the brachioradialis? **Brachioradialis flexes the elbow, and supinates the forearm**

36.   What is the action of the serratus anterior? **Elevates ribs, and protracts and rotates the scapula**

37.   What is the origin of the serratus anterior? **Upper 8 ribs**

38.   What is the insertion of the serratus anterior? **Angles and vertebral border of scapula**

39.   The triceps brachii is the only posterior upper arm muscle which consists of three heads (long, lateral and medial). There are 3 origins. Name these 3 origins. **(1) infraglenoid tubercle of scapula, (2) humerus below radial groove, (3) posterior surface of humerus below great tubercle.**

40.   What are the origins of the posterior, middle and anterior deltoid's and please answer in that order. **Spine of scapula, acromion, lateral clavicle**

41.   What is the action of the peroneus tertius? **Assists in dorsiflexion and eversion of foot**

42.   What is the insertion of the peroneus tertius? **Fifth metatarsal bone**

43.   What is the origin of the peroneus longus? **Upper fibula**

44.   What is the insertion of the peroneus brevis? **Base of the 5th metatarsal bone**

45.   What is the origin of the vastus lateralis? **Linea aspera to greater trochanter**

46.   What is the insertion of the vastus intermedius? **Patella and via patellar ligament to tibial tuberosity**

47.   What is the insertion of the lumbricales manus? **First phalanx and extensor tendon**

48.   What is the action of the abductor pollicis longus? **Abducts and assists in extending the thumb**

49.   What is the action of the gluteus maximus? **Extends and rotates thigh**

50.   What is the origin of the gluteus maximus? **Superior curved iliac line and crest, and sacrum**

51.   What is the insertion of the gluteus minimus? **Greater trochanter**

52.   What is the action of the gluteus medius? **Abducts and rotates the thigh**

53.   What is the origin of the gracilis? **Symphysis pubis and pubic arch**

54. What is the action of the psoas major?   **Flexes thigh, adducts and rotates it medially** What is the insertion of the psoas minor?   **Iliac fascia and iliopectineal tuberosity**

55. What is the origin of the psoas major?   **Last thoracic and all of the lumbar vertebrae**

56. What is the origin of the vastus lateralis?   **Linea aspera to greater trochanter**

57. What is the insertion of the vastus lateralis?   **Common tendon of the quadriceps femoris**

58. What is the action of the vastus lateralis?   **Extends the knee**

59. What is the action of the buccinator?   **Compresses cheek, and retracts angle of mouth**

60. What is the action of the following muscles: Constrictor pharyngis inferior/medius/superior?   **Narrows the pharynx, as in swallowing**

61. What is the origin of the masseter?   **Zygomatic arch and malar process of superior maxilla**

62. What is the action of the mentalis?   **Elevates and protrudes the lower lip**

63. What is the insertion of the mentalis?   **Integument of chin**

64. What is the action of the iliocostalis cervicis?   **Extends cervical spine**

65. What is the origin of the iliocostalis cervicis?   **Angles of 3rd to 6th ribs**

66. What is the action of the iliocostalis lumborum?   **Extends lumbar spine**

67. What is the insertion of the iliocostalis lumborum?   **In angles of 5th to 12th ribs**

68. What is the action of interspinales?   **Supports and extends vertebral column**

69. What is the action of the intertransversarii?   **Flexes vertebral column**

70. What is the action of the rectus capitis posterior major?   **Rotates and draws head backward**
71. What is the origin of the rectus capitis posterior minor?   **Posterior tubercle of atlas**

72. What is the insertion of the rectus capitis posterior major?   **Inferior curved line of the occipital bone**

73.   What is the action of the rectus capitis posterior minor? **Rotates and draws the head backward**

74.   What is the action of the cricothyroideus? **Tightens the vocal cords**

75.   What is the action of the obliquus externus abdominis? **Contracts abdomen viscera**

76.   What is the action of the abliquus internus abdominis? **Obliquus internus abdominus flexes the lumbar vertebral column. Obliquus internus abdominus rotates lumbar vertebral column to the ipsilateral side.**

77.   What is the action of the quadratus lumborum? **Flexes the trunk laterally and forward**

78.   What is the insertion of the quadratus lumborum? **Twelfth rib and the upper lumbar vertebrae**

79.   What is the origin of the coccygeus? **Ischial spine and sacrospinous ligament**

80.   What is the action of the coccygeus? **Supports coccyx, and closes pelvic outlet**

81.   What is the insertion of the coccygeus? **Coccyx and lowest portion of sacrum**

82.   What is the action of the sphincter ani externus? **Closes anus**

83.   What is the origin of the piriformis? **Margins of anterior sacral foramina and great sacrosciatic notch of ilium**

84.   What is the action of the rectus femoris? **Rotates thigh outward**

85.   What is the origin of the rectus femoris? **Iliac spine, upper margin of acetabulum**

86.   What is the insertion of the rectus femoris? **Base of patella**

87.   What is the action of the tensor fasciae late? **Flexes and rotates the thigh**

88.   What is the action of the arrectores pilorum? **Elevates hairs of the skin "goosebumps"**

89.   What is the origin of arrectores pilorum? **Papillary layer of skin**

90.   What is the action of the sternocleidomastoid muscles? **Rotates and depresses the head**

91.   What is the action of the platysma? **Wrinkles skin of neck and chest, and depresses jaw and lower lip**

92.   What is the origin of the medial pterygoid? **Maxilla**

93.   What is the action of the hyoglossus? **Depresses side of tongue and retracts tongue**

94.   What is the action of the salpingopharyngeus? **Elevates nasopharynx (the soft palate)**

95.   What is the insertion of the salpingopharyngeus? **The posterior portion of the pharyngopalatinus**

96.   What is the action of the aryepiglotticus? **Closes glottis opening back of tongue**

97.   What is the insertion of the rhomboids minor? **Proximal portion of spine of scapula**

98.   What is the insertion of the spinalis cervicis? **Axis, and occasionally the two vertebrae below**

End of Muscle Origins and Insertions

99.   What does innervation of muscles mean? **The stimulation of a part of the muscle through the action of nerves or the nerve supply of the muscle.**

100.   What is tissue? **A group or collection of cells which act together in the performance of a particular function**

101.   What are the four primary tissues? **(1) Epithelial (2) Connective (3) muscular (4) nervous**

102.   Name the organs of special sense. **Eyes, Ears, Nose, Tongue, and Skin**

103.   Name the principal systems of the body. **Cardiac, nervous, respiratory, internal secretion, endocrine, skeletal, muscular, reproductive, digestive and, integumentary, lymphatic, and urinary**

104.   What kind of tissue separates the thorax from the abdomen? **Muscle-diaphragm**

105.   What are the most important "tools" of the massage therapist? **Their hands**

106.   Why is the nervous system referred to as the master system of the body? **It is the regulating power in the human body and controls the functions of all organs in the body.**

107.   For purposes of study, anatomists divide the brain into five main parts. Name the parts and indicate which is the largest. **Cerebrum (the**

largest), Cerebellum, The Mid Brain, Pon Varolii, Medula Oblongata

108. Name the two main divisions of the nervous system. **Central nervous system (CNS), peripheral (autonomic nervous system)**

109. What is another name for the central system and peripheral systems? **Voluntary nervous system**

110. How many spinal nerves are found in the normal human body? **31 pair-from vertebrae**

111. What is meant by the statement that the two systems that make up the autonomic nervous system are antagonistic? **One system, the sympathetic, stimulates organs while the parasympathetic depresses the organs functioning**

112. What are the two types of tissue making up the brain, and where is each found? **Gray matter is found on the outer side and the white matter is on the inside**

113. How much bleach solution is used to disinfect? **1:10 ratio i.e. 1 part bleach to 10 parts water**

114. How many years does the IRS require you to keep your records? **7 years**

115. In Chinese medicine what is used for effective digestion? **Ginger, ginseng, and ginkgo**

116. Name the kneading manipulations performed in massage therapy. **Petrissage and friction**

117. Describe the proper friction massage of the upper extremities. **Rolling motion with the palms of hands. In performing the friction manipulations, you should never feel the skin of the client sliding between your hands, but you should feel as though the clients body part is part of your hand, while the muscles and tissues underneath the skin can be felt moving as well as rolling between your palms as you apply the friction manipulations**

118. Describe the therapeutic effect of rolling manipulation massage on the thigh. **Stimulates deep muscles, stimulates nerves and blood circulation**

119. Of what value is knowledge of anatomy and physiology in the profession of massage therapy? **It gives you an overall understanding of the theory behind what you are practicing**

120. Touch that conveys sexuality is considered _____. **Hostile**

121. Define pain. **A subjective experience of the person**

122.   A terminal illness is one where care is _____. **Palliative**

123.   What is diagnosis? **Term used for the signs and symptoms reported by the physician**

124.   When do you have to worry about a mole? **When it changes in color and size**

125.   Why shouldn't you lie on your massage brochures? **It could be misleading and you want to build trust and a respectable practice.**

126.   What movement occurs in the distal radius? **Circumduction**

127.   What is the most common respiratory rate per minute in an elderly patient? **16-25 breaths per minute**

128.   What vessel do you have to be careful of when working the anterior triangle of the neck (an endangerment site)? **Anterior tibial vessels**

129.   What point would you work on for helping to eliminate headaches in Oriental modality? **LI4 is the greatest acupressure point for headaches**

130.   What does the pyloric valve divide? **It divides the mid-intestine from the hind-intestine**

131.   What is "forward head" almost always related to? **Lordosis**

132.   If a patient wants to hug the practitioner after the massage and he/she feels uncomfortable about that, to what code of ethics will these be related to? **Personal boundaries**

133.   When you have to massage a long extremity what is the best posture position? **Put body weight toward the client, using force from the waist**

134.   If someone has low back problems what is the safest way for them to bend? **Bend at the hip and knees**

135.   What is the best way to treat someone with digestive problems? **Light circular motions/abdominal massage helps the movement of food through the ascending and the transverse colons**

136.   What is the name of the action of a muscle that moves the joint to the opposite way from primary movement? **Eccentric**

137.   What muscle is close to the carotid artery? **Sternocleidomastoid**

138.   What is Earth's season? **Late summer**

139.   What is the body's preferred energy source? **Carbohydrates**

140.   What vitamin has to do with the bones and the teeth? **Calcium**

141.   What massage do you do when someone is sensitive to touch? **Reiki**

142.   What provides structure to the body and organs? **Skeletal/Bones**

143.   Two joints that move in a multi-axial plane are _____. **Shoulder and hip**

144.   The chakras are associated with what type of glands? **Endocrine-sensory**

145.   The root chakra is associated with what sense? **Smell**

146.   What organ is NOT associated with Yang? **Liver**

147.   *TRUE OR FALSE.* Massage can activate the lymphatic system? **TRUE**

148.   The hara (the center of gravity) is located where? **Just below the navel**

149.   What action does the triceps brachii perform? **Supination of the forearm at the radioulnar joint.**

150.   What is diverticulitis a disease of? **Large intestine**

151.   The largest artery in the body is_____. **Aorta**

152.   The fight or flight response is controlled by the _____. **Adrenal glands**

153.   The tubes that carry urine from the kidney to the bladder are _____. **Urethras**

154.   What are neurotransmitters? **Chemical messengers**

155.   What hormone does the pineal gland produce? **Melatonin**

156.   The 1099 Tax Form is used to notify the IRS of what information? **Independent Contractor Wages**

157.   What is similar to marmas? **Acupuncture points**

158.   What is most important in taking a Continuing Education   Program? **It must be what is most important to YOU.**

159.   What is Zero balancing? **Zero balancing is a modality that helps relieve physical and mental symptoms; to improve the ability to deal with life stresses; to organize vibratory fields thereby promoting the sense of wholeness and well being.**

160.   What is Somatic Resonance? **It is where the therapist is grounded in their bodily awareness and experience.**

161. What are the most challenging skills in massage? **Listening to our hands while we work and the ability to palpate and respond to the individual tissue variances.**

162. What is Chi Nei Tsang? **A Chinese system of deep healing of the use of energy to the five major systems in the body which are; vascular, lymphatic, nervous, and acupuncture meridians.**

163. Hereditary information is stored in the _____ of a cell. **Nucleus**

164. What connective tissue is strong in all directions? **Dense, irregular, collagen fibers**

165. What is the most common cartilage in the body? **Hyaline**

166. Which layer of the skin acts as an energy storehouse? **Hypodermis**

167. *TRUE OR FALSE.* If your finger is bleeding, you know that the cut is at least as deep as the dermis. **TRUE**

168. What is the most lethal form of skin cancer? **Melanoma**

169. Where are adipose cells found? **In the hypodermis**

170. Which joint is found between the radius and ulna in antebrachium? **Syndesmosis**

171. What are the most common joints found in the body? **Synovial**

172. Fill in the blank by completing the following sequence: abdominal aorta, common iliac artery, _____, femoral artery. **External iliac artery**

173. A deficiency of dietary iodine results in the development of _____. **Thyroid problems**

174. Which movement should be avoided for someone with a hip replacement? **Abduction of the hip**

175. Massage of muscle group would be effective in relieving sciatica? **Gluteus group**

176. What causes poliomyelitis? **A viral infection**

177. *TRUE OR FALSE.* Temporomandibular Joint Dysfunction (TMJ) is a disorder of the mastication muscles and the temporomandibular joints. **TRUE**

178. The mitral valve is also known as the _____. **Bicuspid valve**

179. What are warts? **A contagious infection of the epidermis layer of the skin.**

180.   Proper draping is a very important part of professional business ethics. Why is this so? **It ensures your client's privacy and comfort.**

181.   Which muscle attaches to the zygomatic arch? **Masseter**

182.   Can massage reduce pain and if so, in what way? **Yes. It reduces the cause behind pain stimulation**

183.   When you roll a ball forward on the ground or flat surface, what is the primary movement of the shoulder? **Flexion**

184.   When you stand on your tip-toes your ankle joint goes through _____. **Plantarflexion**

185.   What action are the erector spinae muscles capable of? **Extension**

186.   What muscle of the transversospinalis group is found primarily on the cervical and upper thoracic spine? **Semispinalis**

187.   What type of joint is located between two adjacent vertebrae? **Symphysis**

188.   What is the layer of dense irregular connective tissue that is around all bones? **Periosteum**

189.   *TRUE OR FALSE.* Type I Diabetes Mellitus is characterized by a deficiency of insulin production by thebeta cells within the pancreatic islet cells. **TRUE**

190.   *TRUE OR FALSE.* CST (Cranio Sacral Therapy) works through the crainosacral system to facilitate the performance of the body's inherent self-corrective mechanisms and thereby normalizes the environment in which the central nervous system functions. **TRUE**

191.   How many milligrams of magnesium per day should a massage therapist or anyone else for that matter consume? **400 to 800 milligrams to supplement your diet**.

192.   What are the three steps in helping your clients with chronic pain? **Understand the emotional dimension of chronic pain; help your client realize other healing resources i.e. acupuncture, yoga, etc., and create a safe space so your client feels safe**

193.   *TRUE OR FALSE.* On your intake form referencing pain with 0 being no pain and 10 being worse pain, you could also ask about emotional (psychological) pain? **TRUE**

194.   Name the five types of scars. **Hypertrophie, keloid, trama, surgical, and burn**

195.   What system is the key to restoring muscle memory? **Circulatory system**

196.   What are the two most common joint problems that massage therapists treat? **Osteoarthritis and rheumatoid arthritis**

197.   What are <u>seven steps</u> in <u>setting up a safe and effective</u> work area? **Create comfort by providing all the necessary toiletries, clean sheets, drinking water; make sure the room temperature is comfortable, have controlled lighting, ensure privacy, have a neat treatment room, have a clock in your room that is silent, make sure all equipment is set up properly and in working condition, make the room secure for yourself, as well as for your client**

198.   *TRUE OR FALSE.*   Massage therapist does not have to keep precise records or documentation. **FALSE**

199.   *TRUE OR FALSE.* It is <u>not illegal</u> for a massage therapist to bill for a <u>medical massage</u>. **TRUE**

200.   *TRUE OR FALSE.* Massage therapists can safely and effectively without <u>insurance billing training</u>, bill any insurance companies. **FALSE**

201.   *TRUE OR FALSE.* A massage therapist can not bill higher rates for insurance without repercussion. **TRUE**

202.   *TRUE OR FALSE.* <u>Medicaid</u> will pay a massage therapist. **FALSE**

203.   *TRUE OR FALSE.* A massage therapist can bill an injured worker, in a worker's compensation case, for balances due. **FALSE**

204.   *TRUE OR FALSE.* You do not have to be a "Certified Medical-Massage Therapist" to bill or be reimbursed by insurance. **TRUE**

205.   *TRUE OR FALSE.* If Medicare does not reimburse massage therapists, then insurance companies will follow suit and drop you. **FALSE**

206.   *TRUE OR FALSE.* You can be paid by the supplemental secondary insurance when Medicare is the primary coverage. **FALSE**

207.   In Ayurveda, points are called what? **Marinas**

208.   What is the exercise used to stretch the biceps femoris? **Sit ups**

209.   If you touch the client in an inappropriate sexual way, what is it called? **Hostile**

210.   In psychosomatic theory which region of the body is considered "more male"? **Head and shoulders**

211.   Which is the best way for getting off the massage table after a massage? **Roll to one side with neck relaxed, drop legs off the side of the table, then push up with arms.**

212.   The stomach meridian in relaxation to the body runs in what direction? **Downward**

213.   The therapist drops a pillowcase on the floor, what should be done? **Place in dirty clothes hamper, then wash hands**

214.   Where does the Conception Vessel originate? **Inside of the lower abdomen and emerges from the perineum**

215.   The 3rd chakra color is: **Yellow**

216.   The muscle that abducts the humerus is the _____. **Deltoid**

217.   Which portion of the large intestine passes through the pelvic basin? **Sigmoid**

218.   The client of 50+ years old has a family history of osteoporosis. She wants to prevent it. What exercise might be most helpful? **Weight bearing**

219.   Heavy pressure on the mandible is contraindicated because it could result in what? **Sublimation of jaws**

220.   Which nerve plexus effects anterior arm b/w biceps and triceps? **Brachial**

221.   In massaging biceps femoris, the best position would be with a client in what position? **Prone**

222.   Movement of the body toward the midline is what? **Adduction**

223.   What are the crystallized mineral chunks that develop in the urinary tract called? **Renal Calculi**

224.   What is homeostasis? **It is a state of balance in the body that is maintained through a series of negative feedback mechanisms**

225.   Which muscle groups would you work for lordosis which is same as scoliosis and kyphosis? **Depending on the shape of the curse the therapist would palpate the erector spinae, intercoastals, trapezius and gluteus medius and quadratus lumborum for hypertonicity and trigger points.**

226.   What is the Zygomatic bone? **Cheek bone**

227.   What mineral facilitates actin and myosin? **Adenosine Triphosphate (ATP)**

228.   What is the synergist for the triceps brachia? **Aconeus**

229.   A woman, 40 years old and a survivor of breast cancer can have problems with _____. **(1) bone metrix pericarditis, (2) exophageal efflux, (3) osteomalacia,   and (4) tendon synovitis.**

230.   What is dermatome? **A sensory segment of the skin supplied by a specific nerve root**

231. What is remedial care? **Helps to restore and improve the person's musculoskeletal health**

232. What vitamin is in the eye or what vitamin gel can help the eyes? **Rhodopsin Vitamin A**

233. *TRUE OR FALSE.* Infection can be a response to stress. **TRUE**

234. What exercise is used to stretch the biceps femoris? **Weight training while standing, pace a barbell across the back of your shoulders as you would for squats. Keeping your legs rigid, bend forward at the waist, with head up, until your upper body is parallel with the floor. Reverse the movement to bring your upper body back up.**

235. What do you do with a client that you've been seeing for several sessions who has become repulsive to you lately? **Explain that you do not feel you are helping them and cannot see them anymore. Don't refer them to anybody but suggest they go to a directory to find another therapist.**

236. What taste goes with the spleen? **Sweet**

237. If the medial side of the foot drops what would this be called? **Pigeon toe**

238. If you are in a two-car accident, how would people go about getting the copy of the accident report? **They would get them from the police station once it was reported.**

239. If a client complains of dry eyes and blurry vision, what meridian is out of balance? **Liver**

240. What is the zebra striped pattern called? **A dermatome**

241. The stomach's yin/yang relationship to another organ is? **Spleen (yin)**

242. Mylin is associated with what? **Insulation**

243. Which is distal to the olecranon process? **Ulna**

244. What is Acute Acquired Torticollis and what would be a contraindication with someone who has this? **It is a very painful unilateral shortening or spasm of the muscles in the neck that results in an abnormal head position. Contraindication for any torticolis would be to avoid any full stretches to the sternocleidomastoid muscle and avoid working over the pulse of the carotid triangle immediately anterior to the sternocleidomastoid muscle and inferior to the angle of the mandible.**

245. Why should you not apply deep pressure to the cuboidal area? **Brachial artery**

246. Where does the stomach meridian begin? **Under the pupil of the eye and turns up**

247. Where does the governing vessel originate? **Begins in the pelvic cavity and ascends along the middle of the spinal column to penetrate the brain**

248. The Sciatic nerve passes through which two palpable bony structures? **Hip, and the gluteal region and sometimes through the periformis**

249. What is the name of the muscle that crosses two joints? **Gastrocnemius**

250. How would you position a client with lordosis? **Put a pillow or towel under the belly/tummy to get rid of the exaggeration of the lordotic curve**

251. What kind of fluid would you find in the joints? **Synovial**

252. What would be the best relief treatment for someone with chronic rheumatoid arthritis? **Moist heat**

253. What element would an alcoholic client show in Chinese medicine? **Wood**

254. What type of stretch would you use for joint pain? **Rhythmic initiation stretch**

255. Adult blood cells are made from what? **Red marrow**

256. What is the connective tissue layer covering the entire muscle called? **Epimysium**

257. What is the only bilateral joint? **Saddle joint (the thumb)**

258. What holds the body together? **Fascia**

259. *TRUE OR FALSE.* Homeostasis influences the Endocrine system. **TRUE**

260. *TRUE OR FALSE.* In Chinese medicine, Jing influences the nervous system. **FALSE. The reproductive system.**

261. Yes or No. Both vitamins B and C are water-soluble. **YES**

262. What amino acid breaks down carbohydrates? **Amylase enzyme**

263. What nutrient helps with clotting? **Calcium**

264. What is the action of the masseter muscle? **Elevates the mandible**

265. What is cortisol? **A hormone for the sympathetic nervous system**

266. In Chinese medicine, what is the middle burner? **Digestion**

267.   Name two functions of the circulatory system. **(1) Carries oxygen to the cells of the body, (2) removes waste products from cells of the body**

268.   What system regulates the beating of the heart? **Nervous system**

269.   What is the difference between serum and plasma? **Plasma is the thin yellow liquid portion of the blood that has an anticoagulant, whereas serum has no anticoagulant.**

270.   What are erythrocytes and their function? **Erythrocytes are red blood cells and their function is to carry oxygen and carbon dioxide**

271.   Compare arteries and veins. **Arteries have strong muscular walls consisting of three separate layers. An outer-strong tough layer, a muscular-elastic second layer, and a thin internal coating of connective tissue on the inside. Arteries carry the pure blood from the heart to all parts of the body. Veins are much thinner. They are the "highway" tubes used by the blood.**

272.   What is another word used for applying tapotement? **Percussion**

273.   Why should the massage therapist avoid hacking transversely across the muscle? **May cause a bruise or "Charlie Horse" (a hematoma on the quads caused by a blow).**

274.   How do we govern the amount of pressure used in applying massage? **As much pressure as the client can sand without causing pain, and more pressure to heavily muscled areas.**

275.   Is percussion massage used on the body generally? **No. It is used on the buttocks, thighs, and areas that are heavily muscled at times.**

276.   What is one important physiological effect of tapotement? **Stimulates nerves, restores weak muscles, and is therapeutic.**

277.   What is lymph? **Lymph is a body alkaline transparent colorless fluid found in the lymphatic vessels. It may appear milky in color in vessels draining the intestines because of presence of absorbed fats.**

278.   What moves lymph through the body? **Massage as well as the muscles and joints when they move.**

279.   Does lymph travel through the body as fast as blood? **No**

280.   How is lymph formed? **By plasma and white blood cells escaping through the walls of the capillaries.**

281.   What is the function of the lymphatic system? **Carries digested fats from intestinal area to bloodstream and filters out pus and foreign matter.**

282.   What is meant by the term superficial lymphaticus? **Those near the skin**.

283.   What is the function of the lymphatic valves? **To keep the lymph flowing in one direction**.

284.   What are some of the functions of lymph nodes? **They produce lymphocytes and monocytes and they also will act as filters keeping particulate matter, i.e. bacteria, from gaining entrance to the blood stream**

285.   How is massage helpful in keeping the lymphatic system functioning properly? **It stimulates the flow of lymph.**

286.   What should be the reaction of the client during the massage treatment? **A pleasant relaxed feeling of euphoria**

287.   In what order should massage manipulations be applied in giving a general body massage? **Effleurage, petrissage, friction, tapetoment, and nerve strokes**

288.   Name the three principal classifications of joint movement. **(1) Synarthrosis, amphiarthrosis, and (3) diarthrosis**

289.   Describe one example of each classification. **Synarthrosis— immovable joint—in skull, amphiarthrosis—limited range— spinal column, diarthrosis—freely movable joint—(gliding, hinge, ball and socket joints) wrists and ankles**

290.   Are all joints movable? **NO**

291.   What are the functions of intervertebral discs? **To absorb shock and allow limited movement**

292.   Where is articular fluid found? **In the synovial cavity.**

293.   Define the purpose of articular fluid. **Eliminates much of the friction that would otherwise result when bones are brought in contact with each other during movement**

294.   What is bursa and what is the function of bursa? **Tiny sac sometimes referred to as a "tiny oil can" that is found in all diarthrosis joints, and also found between some of the muscles and underneath some of the muscle structures. The function is to release some of their fluid which acts as a lubricant**

295.   What is meant by sanitation? **Cleanliness**

296.   Why should massage therapists fingernails not extend beyond the pads of their fingers? **So as not to scratch their clients**

297.   *TRUE OR FALSE.* Sanitation in the massage area is good business as well as being healthful for the therapist and the client. **TRUE**

298. Why is knowledge of anatomy necessary before one can become a truly scientific massage therapist? **The massage therapist needs to know the theory behind what they are applying**

299. Name the structures that form the upper extremities. **Shoulders, arms, forearms, and hands**

300. How many bones are found in the upper arm and give their name(s)? **One, Humerus**

301. How many bones are found in the forearm and give their name(s)? **Two, Ulna and Radius**

302. How many bones form the wrist and what are their names? **Eight, They are called carpals**

303. The brachial artery terminates by forming what other arteries? **Radial and ulnar**

304. The radius articulates with what other bones? **The ulna, humerus, for the articulation or hinge joint of the elbow as well as articulation at the wrist**

305. What is the main purpose or function of all muscles in the arm? **Articulation or movement**

306. Why is the triceps muscle so named? **It has 3 heads, or 3 points of contact with bones**

307. If you make a fist with your hands what type of muscles are active flexors or extensors? **Flexors**

308. In massage of the upper limb, what is the first type of manipulation? **Effleurage**

309. In general massage, the manipulations are repeated how many times? **Three**

310. Name the longest bone in the body. **Femur**

311. How many bones are found in the upper leg and give their name(s)? **One, Femur**

312. How many bones are found in the lower part of the leg and give their name(s)? **Two, Tibia and Fibula**

313. How many tarsal bones are found in the normal human body? **14, 7 each Side**

314. Name the largest bone in the lower leg? **Tibia**

315. How many muscles make up the hamstring muscles and give their names? **Three, semimembranous, semitendinous, and biceps femoris**

316.   What is the largest artery in the lower extremities? **Femoral artery**

317.   What are the connecting links between arteries and veins? **Capillaries**

318.   In massage of the lower extremities, the manipulations are applied in what sequence? **Effleurage, tapotement, friction, nerve strokes**

319.   A 76-year-old woman whose frame is small boned and has a history of smoking for many years could possibly develop this. **Osteoporosis**

320.   What causes fascial sheath? **Myofascial**

321.   Why should hacking never be used directly over the tibia? **There is nothing between the tibia and skin**

322.   Tapetoment consists of what five types of manipulation? **Hacking, cupping, tapping, beating with loose fists, and slapping**

323.   Name the main organs located in the thoracic cavity. **Trachea, lungs, esophagus, thymus, and the heart**

324.   What structures join the lungs to the trachea? **Bronchi**

325.   Why is blood in the veins darker than in the arteries? **It contains more waste matter and carbon dioxide**

326.   Name the valves located between the atria and ventricles of the heart. **Tricuspid-the valve on the right side of the heart that has three little flaps, and Bicuspid-the valve on the left side of the heart that has two little flaps**

327.   What are the three steps to help clients navigate through chronic pain? **(1) Understand the emotional dimension of chronic pain, (2) create a safe place for healing, (3) help client to utilize other healing resources**

328.   What two functions are muscle cells limited to? **Contraction and relaxation**

329.   *TRUE OR FALSE.* Music affects no only our minds, but the body as a whole. **TRUE**

330.   What is the perfect posture? **A condition where body mass is evenly distributed and balance is easily maintained during standing and locomotion**

331.   What is the best way to wash your hands? **Use warm running water using liquid plain soap and then dry hands with paper towels**

332.   What are five steps that can be taken to safeguard yourself and your business from lawsuits? **Acceptance, planning, implementation, monitoring, and reaction**

333.   What technique would you use to help alleviate bronchitis symptoms? **Cupping**

334.   *TRUE OR FALSE.* Traditional Thai Massage is shown to reduce pain levels and pain perceptions in patients with non-special low back pain, and then a joint mobilization treatment. **TRUE**

335.   What type of therapy would you suggest for someone who wants to change a movement pattern? **Feldenkrasis**

336.   After changing treatment plans several times without a change in outcome, how would you continue? **Refer person to another professional that could possibly help.**

337.   What type of doctor is trained to treat a subluxation? **Chiropractor**

338.   What does SOAP stand for? **Subjective, Objective, Assessment, Plan**

339.   Name the muscles involved in hip hiking? **Quadratus lumborum**

340.   When should you use CPR? **Cardiac Arrest**

341.   What is the color and organ related to the 4th chakra? **Heart, Green (sometimes pink)**

342.   What does the manual stretching of muscles and fascia create and promote? **Creates mechanical, bioelectrical and biochemical responses that promote improved vascular and lymphatic circulation, increased oxygenation, removal of body toxins and a more efficient nervous system.**

343.   What is one of the reasons for elevating the lower extremity after a strain in acute stage? **To reduce blood flow to the injured areas.**

344.   What should you declare the barter? **100% of the value**

345.   Which muscle is involved in a sciatic nerve pain? **Periformis**

346.   What are the muscles usually involved in shin splint? **Longus muscle and tibialis anterior muscle**

347.   If a marathon runner, after his run, has a high fever, his skin is hot and wet, and his heart rate is high, what is the runner suffering from? **Heat stroke**

348.   At what bony landmark would you locate the kidneys? **12th thoracic**

349.   Which items can be deductible for the IRS? **Business in home**

350.   What color is the chakra for the thyroid? **Sky blue**

351.   Name type of carbohydrate the human body can not digest? **Dietary fiber/cellulose**

352. Which muscles are working when riding a bicycle? **Trunk muscles, Quadriceps**

353. What are the four primary headache types? **(1) Tension,   (2) migraine, (3) Coexisting migraine, and (4) tension-type cluster**

354. What is the first vertebra? **Atlas**

355. If you volunteer at a sports event and work as a massage therapist, what can be deducted on your federal tax return? **Non deductible**

356. When implementing tapping techniques, what specific points are being tapped? **Acupuncture points, chakras, and other energy centers**

357. Why are tapping techniques used? **To move and balance energy in order for the body to heal itself more quickly and effectively.**

358. *TRUE OR FALSE.* Massage therapists should accept tips but not expect them. **TRUE**

359. Where is the best place to palpate the sacrotuberous ligament? **Greater trochanter, lesser trochanter, asis, psis**

360. *TRUE OR FALSE.* Massage therapy helps to decrease blood pressure. **FALSE**

361. What two types of massage affect both diastolic and systolic blood pressure? **Trigger point and sports massage increase both**

362. Where does the heart meridian end? **At the tip of the finger**

363. Where does the lung meridian end? **Corner of base of the thumb nail**

364. What is Zong Qi? **Chinese poetry**

365. What is Zhong Qi? **Chinese calendrics**

366. What is Zhen Qi? **Chinese herbal supplement**

367. What is Wei Qi? **It is the superficial defense energy**

368. Which organs are associated with the metal element? **Lung/large intestine**

369. *TRUE OR FALSE.* The liver and spleen are considered yin. **TRUE**

370. What does the upper burner regulate? **Respiration**

371. Does lymph travel through the body as fast as blood? **NO**

372. Where does the spleen meridian begin? **Medial side of big toe**

373. With which feature is the heart meridian associated? **Tongue**

374.   Which direction does the governing vessel run? **Upward**

375.   An athlete complains of pain the in patella after an event. What would you massage to best help him? **Quadriceps**

376.   What is scar tissue called? **Fibrosis**

377.   How is lymph formed? **By plasma and white blood cells that escape through the walls of the capillaries**

378.   Which hormone is likely to produce pleasure during a massage? **Serotonin**

379.   How would you position a client to stretch the Pectoralis major? **Abduct and laterally rotate the arm**

380.   What is the defining characteristic of rheumatoid arthritis? **Chronic and acute systemic inflammation**

381.   In Western anatomical position, where is the distal ulna? **Medial wrist**

382.   What type of movement does the radioulnar joint have? **Rotation**

383.   What are the five muscles that medially rotate the humerus? **Teres major, anterior deltoid. Subscapularis, pectoralis major, and latissimus dorsi**

384.   Contraction of which muscle can trap the sciatic nerve? **Periformis**

385.   For which condition is moist heat contraindicated? **Edema**

386.   What muscle is associated with spasmodic torticollis? **Sternocleidomastoid**

387.   When palpating the insertion of the illiopsoas muscle, what structure should be avoided? **Femoral nerve**

388.   An injury to one part of the body throws off the entire body. What is this called? **Compensation**

389.   You are massaging a client who begins to have an increased pulse rate and breathing. This likely to be a sign of what? **Anxiety**

390.   Which is an eccentric contraction of the rectus femoris? **Deep knee bends or sit ups**

391.   Give three suggestions you would give a client who has a liver imbalance. **(1) moderate exercise, (2) cut out sweets, fats and alcohol from diet, and (3) small amount of sour in diet**

392.   A supine client you have just finished massaging still has retracted shoulders. Which would you suggest stretching? **Rhomboids**

393.   What is homeostasis? **Relative constancy of the body**

394. *TRUE OR FALSE.* Friction is a contraindication of bursitis. **TRUE**

395. What is the stage that occurs during the first few days of injury, when there is pain, redness, and swelling? **Acute**

396. Two massage therapists decide to work together. What do they have to do to keep their taxes separate? **K-1 form**

397. When is a gift certificate taxable? **When it is purchased**

398. Which involves the inflammation of the tibial tuberosity? **Osgood-Schlatter Disease**

399. What is the best treatment for a client who has chronic constipation and what area would you address? **Use gliding strokes clockwise on the abdomen-stomach**

400. What is the best way to turn a client? **Hold the sheet at the edge farthest from you and have them roll towards you**

401. Is massage indicated for edema? **It is contraindicated. Best to know the difference between edema and lymphedema. Some light massage if legs are eleveated are indicated but you must know the difference between the two before massaging.**

402. What is the term for inflammation of the sheath surrounding a tendon? **Tenosynovitis**

403. Massage may be contraindicated for a client who has_____. **Recent myocardial infarction**

404. Which nerve stems from the brachial plexus? **Radial**

405. A client shows loss of mobility, tension, and elevation in her right shoulder. What could be the possible cause? **Dislocation at the lateral clavicle.**

406. Which hormone is secreted by the pyloric antrium? **Gastrin**

407. What are the most common causes of back pain? **Lumbar strain, nerve irritation, spinal stenosis**

408. What is Spinal Stenosis? **The narrowing of the spinal canal**

409. What regulates the beat of the heart? **The nervous system**

410. What is another word used for applying tapotement? **Percussion**

411. When is gastrocnemius in the isometric position? **In the standing position**

412. How do you massage the quadrates lumborum when your client feels tired and is in the supine position? **Locate the iliac crest anterior to**

posterior go to the 12th rib and do deep muscle on the lateral portion of the quadrates lumborum

413.   What micro nutrient is necessary for hemoglobin? **Iron**

414.   What is probably the symptom or cause of lordosis? **Back pain muscular insufficiency of postural muscles, weak quadrates lumborum**

415.   What nutrient is beneficial for the formation of teeth, bones, the nervous system and aids in sleeping? **Calcium**

416.   The therapist can help the client with scoliosis by doing what? **Compressing the lateral muscles to promote good posture**

417.   Neuromuscular therapy focuses on broad categories of health. Name three. **(1) Biochemistry, (2) biomechanical, and (3) psychosocial influences**

418.   What are the muscles of the rotator cuff? **SITS muscle group (suprapinatus, infrspinatus, teres minor, and subscapularis)**

419.   In Ancient Asian techniques, what is the word for transporting energy Qi? **Meridians**

420.   To palpitate the sciatic notch you would find it where? **Medial gluteus maximus muscle**

421.   How would you work the anterior serratus? **Abduct the arm**

422.   Define neuromuscular therapy. **A comprehensive program of soft tissue manipulation that balances the body's central nervous system with the musculoskeletal system. It is used to evaluate the soft tissues in acute injuries, chronic pain, or dysfunctional patterns of use**.

423.   If a client came in with a recent injury that was red, swollen, and they were in pain, what would you do first? **Apply ice pack**

424.   What structural unit forms all the material in the body? **Cells**

425.   Name at least two functions of the circulatory system. **(1) carries oxygen to the cells of the body and (2) removes waste products from cells of the body**

426.   *TRUE OR FALSE.* The epididymis is part of the male reproductive system. **TRUE**

427.   Where is sperm manufactured? **In the epididymis of the testicles**

428.   Diverticulitis is a disease of the _____. **Large Intestine**

429.   What is a benign effect of prostatic hypertrophy? **Inflammation of the ureters**

430.   What is the sense organ associated with the gall bladder and the liver? **The eyes**

431.   What emotion is associated with the wood element? **Anger**

432.   If a person is laughing uncontrollably and is talking rapidly, what element would they be in excess of? **Fire**

433.   What meridian should not be treated during pregnancy? **SP6**

434.   *TRUE OR FALSE.* Massage should be short in duration and light when working on an infant. **TRUE**

435.   What emotion is associated with the large intestine? **Grief**

436.   What are spinephron and norepinephron secreted from? **Adrenal Medulla**

437.   What is the origin of the gall bladder meridian? **Outer eye**

438.   What chakra is associated with grounding? **Root Chakra (1st)**

439.   What chakra is associated with communication? **The throat (5th)**

440.   What meridian is out of balance if the client has tendonitis? **Liver Meridian**

441.   What insurance protects the massage practitioner/therapist if a client is injured at your office? **General Liability**

442.   *TRUE OR FALSE.* In TCM (Traditional Chinese Medicine) in the initial interview your tongue and pulse are part of the examination? **TRUE**

443.   What muscles are implicated if the shoulder girdle is elevated? **Trapezius and Levator Scapula**

444.   What muscle contracts during inspiration? **Diaphragm**

445.   *TRUE OR FALSE.* The quadriceps eccentrically contract while running down hill to balance the recto abdominus. **TRUE**

446.   Where does conception begin? **Inside the abdomen**

447.   *TRUE OR FALSE.* If the client has extreme kyphosis pillows under the knees would help to lengthen the spine. **TRUE**

448.   *TRUE OR FALSE.* Synovial joints are the most freely moveable joints in the body. **TRUE**

449.   What does endocrine secrete? **Hormones**

450. What organs are protected by sternum and vertebral column? **The heart and lungs**

451. *TRUE OR FALSE.* If a client comes into your office with symptoms of pain down the arm, bluish lips, and shortness of breath, you should immediately call an ambulance. **TRUE**

452. *TRUE OR FALSE.* The actions of the biceps brachii are to flex the elbow and supinate the forearm. **TRUE**

453. At what location is bile emptied into the small intestine? **Duodenum**

454. *TRUE OR FALSE.* Diverticulitis is a disease of the large intestine. **TRUE**

455. *TRUE OR FALSE.* Varices are associated with the respiratory system. **TRUE**

456. What form of draping covers the genitals while enabling access to the rest of the body? **Diaper draping**

457. *TRUE OR FALSE.* When running, heel strike is the point at which the body weight is directly over the leg in contact with the ground. **TRUE**

458. What quadrant ids the liver located? **Upper right quadrant**

459. Name two joints that move in a multi-axial plane? **Knee and shoulder joints**

460. Yes or No. Is the heel referred to as talus? **YES**

461. *TRUE OR FALSE.* A pathway of nerves that is associated with a specific pattern on the skin is called dermatone. **TRUE**

462. *TRUE OR FALSE.* Isometric is when the muscle length stays the same. **TRUE**

463. What is srota? **They are channels or pores according to Ayurvedic Theory**

464. *TRUE OR FALSE.* Massage can activate the lymphatic system. **TRUE**

465. What is the main spinal channel in Ayurvedic medicine? **Sushumna nadi**

466. What is nadi? **They are channels or pathways of energy where prana (ki) flow**

467. Shiatsu is derived from what form of Japanese Massage? **Anma**

468. The water element consists of what yang organ in the five element theory? **The bladder**

469. What is tao? **The law of the universe...also refers to the now, the path or the way**

470. Acupressure points are often referred to as _____.
Tsubos

471. *TRUE OR FALSE.* The kidney is referred to as the foundation of yin and yang of the body. **TRUE**

472. In the five element theory, the _____ element consists of muscles. **Earth**

473. *TRUE OR FALSE.* In the five element theory, the spiritual aspect of water is The Will. **TRUE**

474. *TRUE OR FALSE.* In the five element theory, water element consists of the bladder, a yang organ. **TRUE**

475. *TRUE OR FALSE.* The stomach is associated with the earth element and is referred to as a yang organ. **TRUE**

476. Describe the therapeutic effect of rolling manipulation massage on the thigh. **Stimulates deep muscles, stimulates nerves, and blood circulation**

477. What is located at the base of the spine and is referred to as muladhara? **The root (1st chakra)**

478. What do chakras do? **They are wheels of energy and control the flow of prana (energy)**

479. What element do the heart and small intestine belong to? **The fire element**

480. What element does the trile heater meridian belong to? **The fire element**

481. Where is the greater eliminator (a tsubo) located? **Between the thumb and forefinger**

482. Define pitta. **It is the digestion of food and metabolism of the body and is referred to as "pitta dosha".**

483. What is a dosha? **It is your Ayurveda mind and body type. There are three doshas - vata, pitta, and kappa**

484. Where do you apply moxibustion and what does it look like? **You apply it over the acupuncture points. It looks like a cigar**

485. Name the kneading manipulation performed in massage therapy. **Petrissage and friction**

486. What are some of the functions of the pitta dosha? **It is responsible for digestion conversions, maintains body temperature and hormonal levels, and provides heat and energy to the body, and**

it sharpens intellect and memory, provides color, odor, texture, and luster to the skin.

487.   What is moxibustion? **It is a method of heating by using an herb, artemesia vulgaris**

488.   What gland is the heart chakra associated with? **The thymus gland**

489.   List the seven chakras. **(1) root, (2) sacral, (3) solar plexus, (4) heart, (5) throat, (6) third eye (brow), (7) crown**

490.   In sports and athletic massage, what is defined as "overload"? **Overload can be achieved by manipulating volume and intensity**

491.   What is resistive movement? **It is when the client resists the therapist's movements at the joint, or therapist's resists client's movement**

492.   Muscle fatigue is defined as an inability of a muscle to_____. **Sustain contraction**

493.   What is known as yang or the hollow organ? **The stomach**

494.   Where is the gallbladder meridian located? **Partially located on the lateral aspect of the hip, leg, and foot**

495.   What does Oriental medicine treat? **The Cause**

496.   Tsubos is also known as_____. **Trigger points**

497.   What is the vessel that is a reservoir of yang energy? **Governing vessel**

498.   What is the vessel that is a reservoir of yin energy? **Conception vessel**

499.   What is name of the primary meridian in the back? **The bladder meridian**

500.   Where does the kidney meridian/channel start? **Under the 5th toe and runs to the sole of the foot**

501.   Where does the pericardium channel/meridian start? **It originates from the chest and enters the pericardium, then descends through the diaphragm to the abdomen to communicate with the upper, middle and lower burner**

502.   Where does the liver meridian/channel start? **On the big toe and runs upwards on the dorsum of the foot and medial malleolus, and then up the medial aspect of the leg**

503.   The yin organs store the pure essences resulting from the process of transformation carried out by what? **The yang organs**

504. The five yin organs stores vital substances. What are some of these? **Qi, blood, body fluids, and essence**

505. What is Chi Nei Tsang? **It is a Chinese system of deep healing using the energy of the five major systems in the body which are: vascular, nervous, lymphatic, and acupuncture meridians**

506. *TRUE OR FALSE.* Acupuncture points are similar to marmas? **TRUE**

507. What do the six yang organs do? **They transform and digest**

508. What does yang transform? **Qi**

509. What does yin form? **Structure**

510. Yes or No. Yin and yang are in a constant state of change. **Yes**

511. Name four things in Chinese medicine that constitutes balance. **(1) Sexual life, (2) exercise, (3) Diet, and (4) work**

512. The liver has a couple of functions. What are they? **It stores blood and keeps it moving ensuring the smooth flow of Qi all over the body**

513. What acupuncture point would you use on the lung meridian to reduce a headache? **L14**

514. What are the nine vessels in Oriental medicine? **(1) Governing vessel, (2) Conception vessel (Du Mai), (3) Conception vessel (Ren Mai), (4) Thrusting vessel, (5) Girdle vessel, (6) Yang Hell vessel, (7) Yin heel vessel, (8) Yang linking vessel, and (9) Yin linking vessel**

515. What does the governing vessel control? **It controls all the yang channels**

516. What is the function of the conception vessel? **It monitors and directs all the yin channels including the stomach channel and plays a major role in Qi circulation**

517. What is one of the major purposes of the thrusting vessel? **To connect, communicate and to mutually support the conception vessel**

518. What is considered to be the most vital Yin organ? **The kidney channel**

519. What is the major purpose of the girdle vessel? **To regulate Qi of the gall bladder, and responsible for the strength of the waist area and for the Qi's horizontal balance**

520. *TRUE OR FALSE.* Since a headache is caused by excel Qi (energy) in the head, exercising the legs will draw this Qi downward to the leg muscles and relieve the pressure of the head. **TRUE**

521.   Define meridians. **They are the channels that reach every part of the body and act as the important route for circulating energy and blood**

522.   In TCM (Traditional Chinese Medicine) how does energy flow? **Up and down**

523.   What two systems control homeostasis in the body? **Nervous & Endocrine Systems**

524.   How does governing energy flow? **Base of spine to upper lip**

525.   List the Yin organs according to Chinese medicine. **Kidney, Liver, Heart, Spleen, and Lungs**

526.   What are the five elements in Oriental medicine? **Water, wood, fire, earth, and metal**

527.   Does this female fit the yin or yang? A 35 year old female complains of having (1) no energy, sleeps most of the time if not working, (2) feels cold often and is uncomfortably sensitive to cool environments, (3) skin appears damp, (4) she feels dull emotionally and intellectually, (5) her posture is poor with shoulders that slope forward giving the appearance of a caved-in chest, and (6) when she speaks only her lips move, and she has been having less contact with her friends. **Yin 1**

528.   In TCM there are at least seven commonly used groups of acupoints. What are these points? **Transporting points, five element points, xi-xleft-accumulating points, yuan-source Qi points, mu-front-alarm points, shu-back-points, windows to the sky or heaven**

529.   List the Yang organs according to Chinese medicine. **Gall bladder, small and large intestine, bladder, and stomach**

530.   What is Ayurveda and what makes it unique? **It is a science that is similar to TCM based on individuality of the client which means one particular treatment would not necessarily be right for every client. It uses herbs but no needles like acupuncture.**

531.   What organs are connected to what elements? **Heart-Fire, Stomach-Earth, Lungs-Metal, Kidneys-Water, Liver-Wood.**

532.   Each organ is related to a sense, taste, and emotion. Name all the organs and their corresponding sense, taste, and emotions. **Heart - tongue/speech/bitter taste/joy or hate. Stomach - mouth/lips/sweet taste/worry or peace. Lungs - nose/smell/pungent-spicy taste/grief or courage. Kidneys - ears/hearing/salty taste/ fear or gentleness. Liver- eyes/sight/sour taste/anger or kindness**

533.   How many spinal nerves are found in the normal human body? **31 pair**

534.   Name the five food tastes and give examples of each.   **Hot-ginger, garlic, hot peppers, etc; Warming-potatoes, chicken, honey, cinnamon, etc; Neutral-oats, beets, cabbage, rice, beans, fish, etc; Cooling-barley, mung beans, grapes, mint tea, etc; Cold-melons, cucumbers, pears, tomatoes.**

535.   What chakra is posterior to the scapulae?   **The fourth chakra**

536.   What chakra holds all the energy?   **Every chakra is a wheel of energy**

537.   In TCM, what emotion is associated with wood?   **Anger**

538.   What meridian runs parallel to the spine?   **The urinary bladder meridian**

539.   What percentage of bleach is used to make a disinfectant solution?   **10 parts of water to 1 part bleach**

540.   Define net income.   **Net income is equal to the income after subtracting costs and expenses from the total revenue**

541.   What is the purpose of stretching?   **To improve flexibility and mobility**

542.   *TRUE OR FALSE.* Ligaments connect bone to other bones to form a joint. **TRUE**

543.   *TRUE OR FALSE.* Deep transverse friction is applied in order to reduce adhesions and to help create strong, flexible repair for the healing process. **TRUE**

544.   What is the Golgi tendon organ? **It is a reprioceptive sensory receptor organ that is located at the insertion of skeletal muscle fibers into the tendons of skeletal muscle**

545.   Yes or No. Can a liver be affected in a long-term disease? **YES**

546.   How would you handle a client that shows up for an appointment that is drunk? **Tell them you have to reschedule without offending them**

547.   What hormone activates the sympathetic nervous system? **Central corticotrophin-releasing hormone**

548.   Name some of the benefits/effects of massage on the muscular system. **Improvements in health, such as relaxation or improved sleep, or specific physical benefits, i.e. relief of muscular aches and pains**

549.   *TRUE OR FALSE.* It is okay for the massage therapist to ask a client out on a date. **False, because it violates the "code of ethics".**

550.   *TRUE OR FALSE.* ROM (range of motion) and Touch for Health should never be used to assess a weakness in the muscle. **False, both can assess weaknesses in muscles**

551.   When the therapist assists in the client's ROM, would this be active or passive resistance? **Active**

552.   What nutrient/mineral would help in the formation of bones and teeth? **Calcium**

553.   What part of the body would lordosis be related to? **The back, lumbar**

554.   Yes or No. Lordosis is also referred to as a "curvature of the spine"? **YES**

555.   *TRUE OR FALSE.* Lack of iron in the body is a sign/cause of anemia. **TRUE**

556.   Can hydrotherapy and essential oils have a good effect on the integumentary system? **YES**

557.   What is fascia? **It is a sheath that surrounds muscles, bones, and organs, among several other things in the body**.

558.   What can be some causes of lordosis? **Some muscles around the hip and spine become tight and some become weak. This is due to the position of the tight and weak muscles. Trunk extensors (erector spinae and quadrates lumborum)**

559.   *TRUE OR FALSE.* Hives is a condition that can be contagious from person to person. **FALSE (herpes can be contagious)**

560.   What is another name for a heart attack? **Myocardial infarction**

561.   What is dermatome? **It's a surgical instrument used for cutting thin skin slices for grafting. It also could be the area of the skin supplied by the nerve root, and the lateral part of an embryonic somite.**

562.   What is manible? **The lower jaw**

563.   Name the type of carbohydrate that cannot be digested by humans? **Cellulose**

564.   What type of massage/movement would be best for shoulder pain? **Kneading**

565.   What is another name for ethics? **Moral principles**

566.   What is the first aid for skeletal muscles? **RICE (rest, ice, compression, and elevation)**

567. How many <u>breaths does an adult</u> need per minute under normal circumstances? **14-18 bpm**

568. What (thick muscle) is hard to palpitate in the triangle of the neck? **Sternocleidmastoid**

569. Which one, bronchitis or asthma, has symptoms of wheezing and coughing? **Both**/COPD

570. What is the <u>very first</u> thing a therapist should do if their client is having <u>a seizure</u>? **Hold them and don't put anything in their mouths**

571. Why does cartilage take a log time to heal? **Cartilage in joints is <u>avascular</u>, meaning that it has no direct blood supply. Therefore, nutrients must diffuse to it <u>through the synovial</u> fluid which is slow and inefficient. This slowness causes a slow healing rate.**

572. What two oils should not be used alone when massaging a client? **<u>Essential and mineral oils</u>**

573. Describe a frozen shoulder. **A disorder in which the shoulder capsule, the connective tissue surrounding the glenohumeral joint of the shoulder, becomes <u>inflamed</u> and <u>stiff</u>, and grows together with abnormal bands of tissue, <u>called adhesion</u>, greatly restricting motion and causing <u>chronic pain</u>**

574. Which vitamin has effect on <u>epithelial integrity</u>? **Vitamin A**

575. Define Isotonic. **A muscular contraction in which the muscle remains under relatively constant tension while its length changes**

576. Define Isometric. **A muscular contraction against resistance in which the length of the muscle remains the same**

577. Define Eccentric Contration. **A type of muscle contraction that occurs as the muscle fibers lengthen, such as when a weight is lowered through a range of motion. The contractile force generated by the muscle is weaker than an opposing force, which causes the muscle to stretch**

578. Define Synergist. **A muscle that assists the <u>action of the prime mover</u>**

579. *TRUE OR FALSE.* Paraffin baths are the best use for distal extremities. **TRUE**

580. Define Spina Bifida. **In utero, the <u>two sides of the <u>embryo's spine</u> fail to join together.**

581. Describe why yoga is such an effective modality/practice. **It is gentle, exercises mentally, the mind, and helps you to control the emotion of the body.**

582.   *TRUE OR FALSE.* In general massage the manipulations are repeated 5 times. **FALSE (3)**

583.   When manipulating the upper arm what type of manipulation will you use? **Effleurage**   *stroke*

584.   What is meant by the term superficial lymphaticus? **Near the skin**

585.   What are the functions of the lymph nodes? **Act as filters keeping particular matter, i.e. bacteria, from entering the blood**

586.   The _____ arises from the distal half of the anterior humerus, and inserts upon the coronoid process and tuberosity of the ulna. **Brachialias**

587.   *TERDON*
       TRUE OR FALSE. Aponeurousis is a long flat fibrous membranous sheet that connects a muscle to the bone.   **TRUE**

588.   *TRUE OR FALSE.* The top of the foot only has one muscle, the extensor hallucis longus. It is a thin muscle located between the tibialis anterior and the extensor digitorum longus. It helps to raise the big toe. **TRUE**

589.   *TRUE OR FALSE.* The abductor pollicis brevis abducts the thumb. **TRUE**

590.   *weak*   *Tight*
       TRUE OR FALSE. Gluteus maximus and biceps femoris, hip flexors are the groups of muscles that are involved with extreme lordoris. **TRUE**

591.   Vitamin _____is added to milk. **D**

592.   *TRUE OR FALSE.* Proprioceptors are sensory receptors that are chiefly found in muscles, tendons, joints, as well as the inner ear which detects the motion or the position of the body or a limb by responding to stimuli arising within the organism.   **TRUE** (American Heritage Dictionary)

593.   *TRUE OR FALSE.* The Ileocecal valve is a small muscle. It is located between the small and large intestine and is on the right side of the body. **TRUE**

594.   Yes or No. Should the therapist wait until the sub-acute stage before applying hot moist packs and or ice in an acute inflammation condition? **YES**

595.   *True or False.* Craniosacral therapy is a form of body massage that releases constrictions. It is a manual procedure for remedying distrotionsin the structure and function of the craniosacral mechanism, the brain and spinal cord, the bones of the scull, and it is used to treat chronic pain, migraines, TMJ, sinus pain and other relatated ailments. **TRUE**

596. *TRUE OR FALSE.* Rolfing is a validated system of body restructuring and movement education. It expends less of its vital energies against gravity. **TRUE**

597. *TRUE OR FALSE.* The orbicularis oculi muscle squints the eye. **TRUE**

598. *TRUE OR FALSE.* The golgi tendon organ is a proprioseptive sensory receptor organ transduced by muscle spindles and golgi tendon organs which has compression on the belly of the muscles and the spindle fibers measure tension of the muscles. It is located at the insertion of the skeletal muscle fibers into the tendons of skeletal muscles, being the receptors for stimuli responsible for the lengthening reaction. **TRUE**

599. What are spindle fibers? **They are the structure that separates the chromosomes into the daughter cells**.

600. What is a muscle spindle? **A stretch receptor found in vertebrate muscle.**

601. Yes or No. Is Feldenkrais similar to therapeutic touch? **NO**

602. Is Feldenkrais a deep modality type like rolfing? **NO**

603. If you attend a charity event and you receive tips, what percentage should you report? **All of the money.**

604. *TRUE OR FALSE.* The platysma is a facial muscle attached to the manible. **TRUE**

605. What is cryotherapy and how would a client benefit from it? **It is application of ice, and a client would benefit if they had a torn muscle and if inflammation was present.**

606. In Chinese Medicine, the _____ pulse is used for diagnosis. **The radial pulse**

607. What country is known for creating acupuncture? **China**

608. *TRUE OR FALSE.* Tachycardia is when the heart beats rapidly and the heart pumps less efficiently. **TRUE**

609. *TRUE OR FALSE.* If you have a client who has a condition outside of your SOP, you should refer your client to another physician who has expertise in their condition. **TRUE**

610. Name three places massage therapists can be employed. **(1) Health clubs, (2) Doctors offices i.e. DO's, chiropractor (3) Physical Therapy offices**

611. If you have a client who is looking for energy modalities instead of deep tissue massage, what modality/s would you use? **Therapeutic touch and Reiki**

612. Name fifteen benefits of massage. **(1) increases joint ROM, (2) blood flow, (3) t-cells, (4) flexibility, (5) lymph circulation, (6) promotes healing, (7) hormonal release, (8) homeostasis in sympathetic and parasympathetic systems, (9) improves heart rate and blood pressure,   (10) circulation of oxygen to the cells, (11) improves muscle tone, (12) removes toxins, (13) stretches muscles,   (14) promotes relaxation, (15) reduces pain and stress.**

613. List eight addictions. **(1) sex, (2) food, (3) alcohol,   (4) tobacco, (5) work outs, (6) pain, (7) drugs, (8) drama**.

614. In TCM (Traditional Chinese Medicine) name two organs associated with the earth element.   **Spleen and Pancreas**

615. What two organs are related to the fire element? **Heart and sexual glands**

616. What organ is related to the element of metal? **Lungs**

617. What organ is related to element of water? **Kidneys**

618. What organ is related to the wood element? **Liver**

619. What vitamin would you need if you have anemia? **Vitamin B-12**

620. The _____ controls the flexion of the posterior thigh and leg. **Biceps Femoris**

621. Can you massage a client who has a hernia? **Yes, but not directly on the area.** Compensatry area

622. Are the pectoralis muscles and latissimus dorsi muscles major abductors? **YES** no

623. If you have problems with sciatica, what muscle would be involved? **Piriformis**

624. *TRUE OR FALSE.* The sternoclavicular articulates with the clavicle bone. **TRUE**

625. What are the five abductors of the hip? **(1) Pectineus,   (2) abductor longus, (3) gracilis (4) abductor magnus, (5) abductor brevis**

626. Where is the origin of the five abductors of the hip? **Is on the pubis**

627. *TRUE OR FALSE.* Melatonin and Seratonin are hormones that are produced by the pineal gland. **TRUE**

628. What muscle separates the thoracic cavity from the abdominal cavity? **The diaphragm**

629.   Yes or No. If a client has pain can the therapist determine what might be the problem if they evaluate the gait and the posture of the client. **YES**

630.   *TRUE OR FALSE.* The iliopsoas flexes the hip. **TRUE**

631.   Does the diaphragm relax when inhalation is involved? **No, it contracts during inhalation**.

632.   Yes or No. A goiter is located in the thyroid gland. **YES**

633.   *TRUE OR FALSE.* The popliteal area is an endangered site for the popliteal artery. **TRUE**

628.   *TRUE OR FALSE.* In hydrotherapy the ice pack is used to increase cellular pain. **FALSE, it's used to decrease.**

629.   What is the last part of passage of the colon? **Sigmoid**

630.   What stroke is defined as a slight trembling of the hand? **Vibration**

631.   *TRUE OR FALSE.*   Palpitation is examining with the hands, feeling for organ mass, pulse beat, and sense of touch. **TRUE**

632.   *TRUE OR FALSE.* Radioulnar joints roatate. **TRUE**

633.   When you are massaging the upper aspect of the pectoral what endangerment site is involved in that area? **Subclavin artery**.

634.   *TRUE OR FALSE.* The biceps brachi is attached to the caracoid process. **TRUE**

635.   What does protraction do to the muscle? **It lengthens it**

636.   What endangerment site is on the C1 and C4? **Cervical plexis**

637.   *TRUE OR FALSE.* If abduction of the lateral rotators occurs, the piriformis muscle is contracted. **TRUE**

638.   *TRUE OR FALSE.* The levator scapula is involved if the scapula is elevated. **TRUE**

639.   Define what universal precaution does. **Prevents the spread of diseases**.

640.   Purple spider like veins, also blue, raised, and bulging veins are an indication of_____. **Varicose veins**

641.   *TRUE OR FALSE.*   Deep breathing is the best form of relaxation for both the client and the therapist. **TRUE**

642.   *TRUE OR FALSE.*   Urine goes through the urethra after it passes through the bladder. **TRUE**

643.   Where is the phrenic nerve located? **The posterior nerve of the neck.**

644.   Define metabolism. **The process that breaks down the food we eat.**

645.   Define carrier oil. **It is oil that is mixed with essential oils.**

646.   What does the perimysium, epimysium, and endomysium cover? **Muscle**

647.   Give a few reasons why you would use light massage on the face. **Sensitive areas, little depth of muscle, delicate muscle tissue, nerves and arteries close to the surface.**

648.   *TRUE OR FALSE.* Active herpes is locally contraindicated. **TRUE**

649.   *TRUE OR FALSE.*   Ringworm is a fungus and can be spread by a dog. **TRUE**

650.   Define SOP (Scope of Practice). **Relates to skills and training received also described in a legal description and definitions contained in licensing regulations.**

651.   *TRUE OR FALSE.*   When the right shoulder is lifted the upper trapezius muscle is activated. **TRUE**

652.   Name the two muscles of the iliopsoas. **Psoas major and iliacus**

653.   *TRUE OR FALSE.* You have a client on the table and you notice they are extremely thin and loosing hair and you have reason to believe your client is anorexic. You would bolster your client and proceed with the massage cautiously. **TRUE**

654.   *TRUE OR FALSE.* If a client is supine and the femur is abduct the hip, the tensor faciae latae muscle will shorten. **TRUE**

655.   *TRUE OR FALSE.* The number 10 cranial nerve passes through the neck and thorax into the abdomen and supplying sensation to part of the ear, the tongue, the larynx, and the pharynx, motor impulses to the vocal cords, and motor and secretory impulses to the abdominal and thoracic visceracranial nerves, innervates abdomen and thoracic viscera. **TRUE**

656.   Where are the Islets of Langerhans found? **The pancreas**

657.   In what order does food pass through the small intestine during digestion. **First the duodenum, second jejunum, and last the ileum.**

658.   Is areolar an epithelial tissue? **No, it's is loose connective tissue. It binds skin to underlying tissues and fills spaces between muscles. It is also known as superficial fascia.**

659.   *TRUE OR FALSE.* The knee is proximal to the foot. **TRUE**

660.   *TRUE OR FALSE.* The cells of the liver do not detoxify poisons.
FALSE. They do detoxify poisons.

661.   *TRUE OR FALSE.* The quadratus lumborum is the muscle that holds
down the twelfth rib on respiration. **TRUE**

662.   _____ _____ are the muscles that have the opposite
functions? **Antagonistic muscles**

663.   Name three of the dense connective tissues.
Tendons, ligaments, and joint capsules.

664.   _____ _____ is the name of the spongy layer just below the
skin? **Superficial Fascia**

665.   How do you differentiate superficial fascia from muscles?
**Pick up the skin and the superficial fascia, and then contract
the underlying muscles**.

666.   What is Orthopedic Massage? **Techniques for understanding,
assessing, and treating musculoskeletal pain and injury.**

667.   What is found directly under superficial fascia and what does it cover?
**Deep Fascia. It covers all the muscles and bones blending into
ligaments and joint capsules and wrapping organs.**

668.   *TRUE OR FALSE.* Most cases of muscle spasms are actually the result
of injury to some other tissue. **TRUE**

669.   *TRUE OR FALSE.* Muscles are a major source of pain and injury.
FALSE

670.   *TRUE OR FALSE.* Chronic pain results when an injury heals improperly.
TRUE

671.   What is secreted by the ovaries? **Estrogen**

672.   Where does the conception vessel start? **Peritoneum**

673.   The _____ system is responsible for the cardiovascular blood
flow? **Lymphatic**

674.   Ki 1 is found where on the body? **Sole of the foot**

675.   Would you perform massage if the client has Thrombophlebitis? **NO**

676.   Is the Meisner Corpuscle sensitive to touch? **YES**

677.   What gland is associated with the third eye chakra? **Pineal**

678.   What would be out of balance in the wood element? **Sight**

679.   *TRUE OR FALSE.* You should never lie on your massage brochures

because you want to build trust with your clientele. **TRUE**

680.   _____ _____ is *extreme* inflammation of the
joints. **Rheumatoid arthritis**

681.   *TRUE OR FALSE.* When a client tells you they have an eating disorder,
you must keep it confidential. **TRUE**

682.   St 36 is on what part of the body? **Anterior calf**

683.   In the 5-Element Theory, the _____ spreads pain to other areas
of the body.   **Wind**

684.   Where would you place a pillow if a client has back and hip pain? Under
the legs behind the knees.

685.   In Ayurvedic medicine, energy fields are called _____.
Doshas

686.   Why is taking a Continuing Education Program important? You are

learing something new to improve your professional development.

687.   What is the most common pulled muscle and how would you treat it?
**Hamstring and you would treat it via R.I.C.E. Rest, Ice,
Compressin, and Elevation**

688.   What sense organ is associated with water? **Ears**

689.   What is the most water repellent part of the body? **The skin**

690.   What is connected to the hypothalamus? **Pituitary Gland**

691.   *TRUE OR FALSE.* In many cases pain is *referred* from the source of
energy to another part of the body. **TRUE**

692.   What does the spleen nourish? **Lungs**

693.   The three functions of the blood are to _____,
_____ and _____.
Nourish the body, moisten the body and aid the mind.

694.   In Traditional Chinese Medicine, Qi has four directions. They
are _____, _____, _____ and
_____. **Ascending, descending, entering and
leaving.**

695.   *TRUE OR FALSE.* A woman who had chemotherapy for breast cancer 8
years ago could still have dark areolas. **TRUE**

696.   What does histamine do? **It contributes to an inflammatory response and causes constriction of smooth muscle.**

697.   Define Holistic Health. **It is medical care involving the treatment of the whole person – Body/Mind/Spirit.**

698.   *TRUE OR FALSE.* The shoulders, neck, thorax, lower back, sacrum, buttocks and hip joints are the only significant sources of referred pain. **TRUE**

699.   If you are working on a client who has problems with TMJ what muscles would you work on? **The pterygoids and the masseter mussles**

700.   If a client has PTSD (Post-Traumatic Stress Disorder) and just found out they had been sexually abused, what would be the best recommendation for you to do? ___. **Refer them to a psychotherapist.**

701.   What is Flexion-Addiction and what does it promote?
It is prolonged sitting due to being a couch potato, sitting long hours at a computer, or sleeping in a flexed position. It promotes length tension, imbalances resulting in tight/short hip flexors and neurologically weakened hip extensors.

702.   What protein would the body rather have as use for energy? **Protein! (A protein does not go by another name) Watch out for trick questions on exams.**

703.   The _____ and _____ _____ muscles are shortened due to prolonged sitting and sleeping. **Iliopsoas and rectus femoris**

704.   If someone has a seizure, what would you do? **Stay calm and make sure the area is safe so the person will not be injured. Stay with the person until the seizure passes.**

705.   When someone has gout, the mineral _____ is lacking. **Calcium**

706.   The part of the colon that passes through the pelvic outlet is the _____. **Sigmoid**

707.   How do you stretch pectoralis major? **Stand at the end of a wall or in doorway facing perpendicular to wall. Place inside of bent arm on surface of wall. Position bent elbow at shoulder height. Turn body away from positioned arm. Hold stretch. Repeat with opposite arm.**

708.   What taste is associated with the spleen? **Sweet**

709.   The _____ (organ) is located posterior to the xiphoid process. **Liver**

710.   Where are plantar warts located? **On the soles of the feet**

712.   If a client has constipation, you would first massage the
_____. **Abdomen**

713.   *TRUE OR FALSE.* Pain caused by active movements gives a good
indication of what structure is injured.   **FALSE**

714.   What is ischemia? **It is a lack of oxygen to the muscles**

715.   What is Somatic Resonance? **It is the therapist being grounded in
their bodily awareness and experience.**

716.   By shortening the rectus femoria what exercise will it perform? **Knee
extension and hip flexion**

717.   When you are performing ROM and come across resistance, what do
you do? **You stop.**

718.   _____ tissue covers all organs. **Epithelial**

CPR 719.   When _____ you should stop giving resuscitation.
Breathing returns

720.   The kidney is associated with the _____ chakra. **6th**

721.   The 3rd chakra is associated with what pair? **Solar plexus/navel -
Action and Will**

722.   Visceral is part of the _____ system. **Autonomic
system, which is part of the parasympathetic system**

723.   Where does the heart meridian begin? **Under the arm**

724.   Where does the heart meridian end? **At the little finger**

725.   Where do you find the sciatic notch? **L5 S1**

726.   What are ethics?
Motivations based on ideas of right and wrong

727.   _____ _____ and _____ are associated with the bladder?
Urine storage and output

728.   When flexing the elbow, what muscle is involved?
Brachioradialis

729.   Study this chart.

Element	Color	Organ/s	Sense Organs	Taste
Water	Black	Kidneys/Bladder	Ears	Salty
Wood	Blue/Green	Liver/Gall Bladder	Eyes	Sour
Fire	Red	Heart/Small Intestine	Tongue	Bitter
Earth	Yellow	Spleen/Stomach	Mouth	Sweet
Metal	White	Lungs/Large Intestine	Nose/Sinuses	Spicy

730.   Sea water on the earth would be like _____ in the human because they both have a narrow pH range.   **Blood**

731.   Where do you find pulmonary semilunar valve? **It lies between the right ventricle and the ulmonary artery and has three cusps**

732.   What gland is associated with heart chakra?   **Thymus gland**

733.   Parkinson's disease may start with a slight _____. **tremor**

734.   _____ _____ is synergist to periformis.
        Gluteus maximus

735.   In a client who has kyphosis,(another name for this is Dowager's hump) what muscle would you suggest they stretch? **Pectoralis**

736.   The _____ _____ muscle is involved in flexing the forearm.
        Biceps brachii

737.   In Oriental Medicine, Yang channel flows in what direction?
        Down

738.   Where is the sperm manufactured?
        In the testes. It is matured and stored in the epididymis, which is part of the male reproductive system.

739.   The function of the Lung Meridian is to _____
        _____.
        govern the respiratory system, skin, perspiration, and energy and body temperature regulation.

740.   A client comes into your office and is having pain when trying to put on a shirt or coat. What muscle is causing the problem? **Rhomboids and supraspinatus**

741.   The _____ _____ and the _____ are two muscles that don't tire easily. **Rectus Femoris and Periformis – (smooth muscles)**

742.   What is Ischemia? **Decreased blood flow**

743.   What is the sense organ associated with the gall bladder and liver?
        Eyes

In Chinese medicine emotions are associated with certain organs. Be sure and study the below list.[1]

SPLEEN

Emotions - worry, dwelling or focusing too much on a particular topic, excessive mental work

Spleen Function - Food digestion and nutrient absorption. Helps in the formation of blood and energy. Keeps blood in the blood vessels. Connected with muscles, mouth, and lips. Involved in thinking, studying, and memory.

Symptoms - of Spleen Imbalance - Tired, loss of appetite, mucus discharge, poor digestion, abdominal distension, loose stools or diarrhea. Weak muscles, pale lips. Bruising, excess menstrual blood flow, and other bleeding disorders.

LUNG

Emotions - grief, sadness, detached.

Lung Function - Respiration. Forms energy from air, and helps to distribute it throughout the body. Works with the kidney to regulate water metabolism. Important in the immune system and resistance to viruses and bacteria. Regulates sweat glands and body hair, and provides moisture to the skin.

Symptoms - of Lung Imbalance - Shortness of breath and shallow breathing, sweating, fatigue, cough, frequent cold and flu, allergies, asthma, and other lung conditions. Dry skin. Depression and crying.

LIVER

Emotions - anger, resentment, frustration, irritability, bitterness, "flying off the handle."

Liver Function - Involved in the smooth flow of energy and blood throughout the body. Regulates bile secretion, stores blood, and is connected with the tendons, nails, and eyes.

Symptoms of Liver Imbalance - breast distension, menstrual pain, headache, irritability, inappropriate anger, dizziness, dry, red eyes and other eye conditions, tendonitis.

HEART

Emotions - lack of enthusiasm and vitality, mental restlessness, depression, insomnia, despair.

Heart Function - Regulates the heart and blood vessels. Responsible for even and regular pulse. Influences vitality and spirit. Connected with the tongue, complexion, and arteries.

Symptoms of Heart Imbalance - Insomnia, heart palpitations and irregular heart beat, excessive dreaming, poor long-term memory, psychological disorders.

KIDNEY

Emotions - fearful, weak willpower, insecure, aloof, isolated.

Kidney Function - Key organ for sustaining life. Responsible for reproduction, growth and development, and maturation. Involved with lungs in water metabolism and respiration. Connected with bones, teeth, ears, and head hair.

Symptoms of Kidney Imbalance: Frequent urination, urinary incontinence, night sweats, dry mouth, poor short-term memory, low back pain, ringing in the ears, hearing loss, and other ear conditions. Premature grey hair, hair loss, and osteoporosis.

[1]**. Thanks to Cathy Wong for the information listed above.**

744.   What emotion is associated with the kidneys and bladder? **Fear**

745.   What composes the Autonomic Nervous System? The sympathetic and the parasympathetic systems.

746.   _____ is excess fluid build-up in the tissues. **Edema**

747.   If a new client is hesitant about filling out an intake form, you should _____. **Ask them the questions and write down what they tell you.**

748. The _____ is an example of a Yin Organ. **Liver**

749.   A client wants to give you a hug after a massage session and you do not feel comfortable. This is an example of _____. **Personal boundaries**

750. When a physician writes out a "comfort order" it is usually done for this type of patient. **Terminally ill patient**

751.   What emotion is associated with the wood element? **Anger**

752.   The kneecap is also called the _____. **Patella**

753.   The collar bone is also called the _____. **clavicle**

754.   The thigh bone is also called the _____. **femur**

755.   _____ and _____ are comprised primarily of dense fibrous tissue. **Tendons/ligaments**

729.   Study this chart.

Element	Color	Organ/s	Sense Organs	Taste
Water	Black	Kidneys/Bladder	Ears	Salty
Wood	Blue/Green	Liver/Gall Bladder	Eyes	Sour
Fire	Red	Heart/Small Intestine	Tongue	Bitter
Earth	Yellow	Spleen/Stomach	Mouth	Sweet
Metal	White	Lungs/Large Intestine	Nose/Sinuses	Spicy

730.   Sea water on the earth would be like _____ in the human because they both have a narrow pH range.   **Blood**

731.   Where do you find pulmonary semilunar valve? **It lies between the right ventricle and the ulmonary artery and has three cusps**

732.   What gland is associated with heart chakra?   **Thymus gland**

733.   Parkinson's disease may start with a slight _____. **tremor**

734.   _____ _____ is synergist to periformis.
Gluteus maximus

735.   In a client who has kyphosis,(another name for this is Dowager's hump) what muscle would you suggest they stretch? **Pectoralis**

736.   The _____ _____ muscle is involved in flexing the forearm.
Biceps brachii

737.   In Oriental Medicine, Yang channel flows in what direction?
Down

738.   Where is the sperm manufactured?
In the testes. It is matured and stored in the epididymis, which is part of the male reproductive system.

739.   The function of the Lung Meridian is to _____
_____.
govern the respiratory system, skin, perspiration, and energy and body temperature regulation.

740.   A client comes into your office and is having pain when trying to put on a shirt or coat. What muscle is causing the problem? **Rhomboids and supraspinatus**

741.   The _____ and the _____ are two muscles that don't tire easily. **Rectus Femoris and Periformis – (smooth muscles)**

742.   What is Ischemia? **Decreased blood flow**

743.   What is the sense organ associated with the gall bladder and liver?
Eyes

772.   The _____ chakra, which is associated with communication, is the _____ (number) chakra. **Throat/5th**

773.   Energy fields in Ayurvedic medicine are called _____. **Meridians**

774.   What meridian is out of balance if the client has tendonitis? **The liver meridian**

775.   In TCM (Traditional Chinese Medicine), the 4 examinations occur_____. **At the initial interview.**

Of Interest

There are four examination methods: Questioning/history taking, inspection, auscultation (listening) & olfaction (smelling), and palpation. The four methods have their unique clinical functions and cannot be replaced by one another. Sometimes, false manifestations of a disease occur which emphasize the importance of integrating all diagnostic methods.

776.   *TRUE OR FALSE.* The gluteus maximus extends and laterally rotates the thigh. **TRUE**

777.   TRUE OR FALSE. During downhill running, your quadriceps muscles contract eccentrically to resist the pull of gravity. **TRUE**

778.   *TRUE OR FALSE.* The Conception Vessel starts from the inside of the abdomen and emerges from the perineum. **TRUE**

779.   Some joints have more Range of Motion than others. Which joint would have the most ROM? **Diarthrosis**

780.   What are the most freely movable joints in the body? **Synovial Joints**

781.   What do endocrine glands secrete? **Hormones**

782.   The tubes that carry urine from the kidney to the bladder are called_____. **Ureters**

783.   _____ attaches muscles to bones. **Tendons**

784.   What does the trunk of the body refer to? **The chest and the abdomen.**

785.   What is the purpose of the lymph system? **It is responsible for fighting disease and infections.**

786.   *TRUE OR FALSE.* A musculotendinous strain is indicated if resisted joint motion reproduces the complaint. **TRUE**

787.   What is an impacted fracture? **A fracture is an injury to a bone when the tissue of the bone is broken**

788. A 62 year old man comes to your office with pain down his left arm, bluish lips, and shortness of breath. You should immediately _____. **Dial 911**

789. What is the action of the biceps brachii? **Turns the palm upward.**

790. Where does the bile duct lead? **From the gallbladder and liver into the duodenum**

791. What is another name for a heart attack? **Myocardial infarction**

792. What structures join the lungs to the trachea? **Bronchi**

793. What muscle separates the abdomen from the thorax? **Diaphragm**

794. When you stop performing ROM and come across resistance what do you do? **Stop**

795. Where are plantar warts located? **On the soles of feet**

796. What does the spleen nourish? **Lungs**

797. Is the Meisner Corpuscle sensitive to touch? **Yes**

798. True or False. Muscles are a major source of pain and injury. **TRUE**

799. Should massage ever cause your client discomfort? **NO**

800. _____ is needed to strengthen bones, provide muscle contracture. **Calcium**

801. The hip area is in what section of the body? **It is in the gluteal section.**

802. _____draping covers the genitals while enabling access to the rest of the body. **Diaper**

803. Is Chiropractic subluxation the same as medical subluxation? **NO**

804. Yes or No. You should be careful in movements of the joints with the elderly. **YES**

805. True or False. The major muscle of cheek is the buccinator. **TRUE**

806. Could a client faint is you press to hard and long on the carotid artery. **YES**

807. What does B1 stand for? **Bladder Meridian**

808. True or False. The lympathatic system drains in the subclavian vein. **TRUE**

809.   When running, the point at which the body weight is directly over the leg in contact with the ground is _____. **Mid-stance**

810.   The liver is located in the_____. **Upper right quadrant of the abdomen.**

811.   Can CE (Continuing Education) be deducted from your expenses on Tax Forms?   **YES**

812.   What is another name for the cervical region?   **Mesenchephalon**

813.   The heel bone is the_____.   **Calcaneus**

814.   During treatment, a client who starts to breathe more rapidly may be experiencing_____.   **Anxiety**

815.   A pathway of nerves associated with a specific pattern on the skin is called a _____.   **Meridian**

816.   You come across a scene with an apparently unconscious person. Your first step should be to _____.   **Check for responsiveness.**

817.   Which receptors sense deep touch?   **Golgi tendon receptors**

818.   The muscle action in which the muscle length stays the same is_____.   **Isometric**

819.   During the client interview, if the therapist was leaning back in a chair with her arms and legs crossed would this send a 'message' that the therapist was not very interested in their work?   **YES**

820.   A doctor might recommend massage for a cancer patient to: **Provide comfort and stress reduction**

821.   The best way to treat bursitis is with an _____?   **Ice pack**

822.   When you laterally rotate the femur, what muscle shortens? **Piriformis**

823.   What is diagnosis?   **Term used for the signs and symptoms reported by the physician.**

824.   Name the movement that occurs in the distal radius?   **Flexion**

825.   Name primary function of pain?   **Warns you of tissue damage**

826.   What point would you work on for headaches in TCM modality?   **GV 19/20 Governing Vessel 19**

827.   What does the pyloric valve divide?   **It divides the mid-intestine from the hind-intestine**

828.   Yes or No.   Is forward head related to Kyphosis and lordosis?   **YES**

829. If a patient wants to hug the practitioner after the massage and he/she feels uncomfortable about that, to what code of ethics will these be related to?   **personal boundaries**

830. When you have to massage a long extremity what is the best posture position? **The Horse Stance**

831. What is the best way to treat someone with digestive problems? **Effleurage in the abdominal area**

832. What is the name of a muscle that moves the joint to the opposite way from primary movement? **Antagonist**

833. What muscle is close to the carotid artery? **Sternocleidomastoid**

834. What is Earth's season?   **Late Summer**

835. Name the body's preferred energy source? **Carbohydrates**

836. What vitamin helps the bones and the teeth**?   Calcium**

837. What type of massage do you do when someone is sensitive to touch? **Reiki**

838. Name the technique that involves pumping _____. **Compression**

839. Name what provides structure to the body and organs. **Skeletal /bones**

840. To assess a client's ROM what series would you put them through? **Joint mobilization**

841. Name 2 joints that move in a multi-axial plane. **Shoulder & hip**

842. What type of glands are the charkas ssociated with? **Endocrine-sensory**

843. The first chakra (root chakra) is associated with what sense?   **Smell**

844. Is liver associated with Yang**?   NO**

845. Can massage activate the lymphatic system? **YES**

846. Where is hara, which is the center of gravity located?   **Just below the navel**

847. Does the triceps brachii perform supination of the forearm at the radioulnar joint? **YES**

848. Is diverticulitis a disease of the Large intestine? **YES**

849. What is the largest artery in the body? **The Aorta**

850.   What controls the fight or flight response? **The Adrenal Glands** *symputufies. N*

851.   What carries the urine from the kidney to the bladder? **The Urethras**

851.   Define neurotransmitters? **They are Chemical messengers**

852.   What is the hormone the pineal gland produces?   Melatonin

853.   What is the 1099 Tax Form used for. **To report Independent Contractor Wages to the IRS**

854.   Why is taking a Continuing Education Program important? **You are learning something new to improve professional development**

855.   What is Zero Balancing? **Zero Balancing is a modality that helps relieve physical and mental symptoms; to improve the ability to deal with life stresses; to organize vibratory fields thereby promoting the sense of wholeness and well being.**

856.   What is Somatic Resonance? **It is where the therapist is grounded in their bodily awareness and experience.**

857.   What is a most challenging skill in massage? **listening to our hands while we work and the ability to palpate and respond to the individual tissue variances (assessment)**

858.   List three causes of disease. **Stress, trauma, & malnutrition**

859.   Define Chi Nei Tsang?   **A Chinese system of deep healing of the use of energy to the five major systems in the body which are: vascular, lymphatic, nervous, and acupuncture meridians.**

860.   What is like marmas? **Acupuncture points**

861.   Where is hereditary information stored? **In the Nucleus**

862.   Name the connective tissue that is strong in all directions? **Dense, irregular, collagenous connective tissue**

863.   Name the most common cartilage in the body? **Hyaline**

864.   Name the layer of the skin that acts as an energy storehouse? **Hypodermis**/ *Fat*

865.   TRUE OR FALSE. If your finger is bleeding, you know that the cut is at least as deep as the Dermis.   **TRUE**

866.   Name the most lethal form of skin cancer? **Melanoma**

867.   Name location on body where adipose cells are found? **In the hypodermis**

868.   Name the joint that is found between the radius and ulna in the antebrachium? **Syndesmosis**

869.   Name the most common type of joint found in the body? **Synovial**

870.   TRUE OR FALSE. A goiter results from a deficiency of dietary iodine. **TRUE**

871.   Name the movement that should be avoided for someone with a hip replacement? **Abduction of the hip**

872.   What group of muscles would you massage that would help to relieve sciatica? **Gluteus group**

873.   What caused poliomyelitis? **A viral infection**

874.   What is another name for the mitral valve? **Bicuspid valve**

873.   Define what warts are. **A contagious infection of the** epidermis layer of the skin

874.   Why is proper draping an important part of professional business ethics? **It ensures your client's privacy and comfort**

875.   Name the muscle that attaches to the zygomatic arch? **Masseter**

876   Can massage reduce?   **YES**

877.   If you are rolling a bowling ball forward, what is the primary movement of the shoulder? **Flexion**

878.   While standing on your tip-toes your ankle joint goes through_____. **Plantarflexion**

879.   Name the action the erector spinae muscles are capable of? **Extension**

879.   Name the muscle of the transversospinalis group ithat is found primarily on the cervical and upper thoracic spine? **Semispinalis**

880.   Name the type of joint that is located between two adjacent vertebrae? **Symphysis**

881.   TRUE OR FALSE. Periosteum is the layer of dense irregular connective tissue that is around all bones. **TRUE**

882.   Is Type I Diabetes Mellitus characterized by a deficiency of insulin production by the beta cells within the pancreatic islet cells. **YES**

883.   Define CST (CranioSacral Therapy). **CST works through the crainosacral system to facilitate the performance of the body's inherent self-corrective mechanisms and thereby normalizes the environment in which the central nervous system functions.**

884.   TRUE OR FALSE. 400 to 800 milligrams of magnesium should be taken every day to supplement your diet. **TRUE**

885.   List three steps in helping your clients with chronic pain? **Understand the emotional dimension of chronic pain; help your client realize other healing resources i.e. acupuncture, yoga, etc.; and create a safe space so your client feels safe, learn body language, move slowly, respect the boundaries of the client and don't impose your own ideas of what the session should be like.** Also: List at least four types of scars. **Hypertrophic, keloid, trama, surgical, and burn**

886.   What are some of the things you should be aware of that fall into the category of Boundaries? **Don't criticize someone's belief systems, don't have any sexual relationships with clients, be aware of the emotional and mental states of your clients and don't reveal your feelings or talk about personal issues with a client and dress appropriately during a session.**

887.   What are some of the various types of insurance coverage?

**Small Business Insurance
Product Liability
Personal Disability Insurance
Malpractice Liability Insurance
General Liability Insurance
Workers Compensation**

Name some steps in setting up a safe and effective work area? **Create comfort by providing all the necessary toiletries i.e. clean sheets, drinking water, make sure the room temperature is comfortable, have controlled lighting, ensure privacy, have a neat treatment room, have a clock in your room that is silent, make sure all equipment is set up properly and is in working condition, make the room secure for yourself, as well as for your client.**

888.   Does the nervous system include the brain? **YES**

890.   TRUE OR FALSE. A massage therapist can accept any type of insurance case. **FALSE**

891.   TRUE OR FALSE. As a massage therapist I do not have to keep precise records or documentation. **FALSE**

892.   Two True of False's. A massage therapist can not bill higher rates for insurance without repercussion. **TRUE.** It is not illegal for a massage therapist to bill for a medical massage. **TRUE**

893.   True of False. Medicaid will pay a massage therapist. **FALSE**

894.   True of False. A massage therapist can bill an injured worker, in a worker's compensation case, for balances due. **FALSE**

895.   TRUE OR FALSE. You do not have to be a "Certified Medical-Massage Therapist" to bill or be reimbursed by insurance. **TRUE**

896.   TRUE OR FALSE. If Medicare does not reimburse massage therapists, then insurance companies will follow suit and drop you. **FALSE**

897.   What does GB in Oriental Medicine mean? **Gall Bladder**

898.   How would you relieve pressure on the lower back? **Putting a support under the ankles.**

899.   TRUE OR FALSE. You can be paid by the supplemental / secondary insurance when Medicare is the primary coverage. **FALSE**

900.   In Ayurveda, points are called what? **Marmas**

901.   Name the exercise used to stretch the biceps femoris? **Sit ups**

902.   If you touch the client in a sexual way, what is this called? **Hostile**

903.   In psychosomatic theory what region of the body is considered *more male*? **Head and shoulders**

904.   What is the best way to get off of the massage table after a massage? **Roll to side with neck relaxed, drop legs off the side of table, then push up with arms.**

905.   What direction does the stomach meridian run? **Downward**

906.   If the therapist drops a pillow case on the floor, what should they do? **Place in dirty clothes hamper, then wash hands**

907.   Where does the Conception Vessel originate? **Inside of the lower abdomen and emerges from the perineum**

908.   What is the 3rd charka color? **Yellow**

909.   Name the muscle that abducts the humerus. **Deltoid**

910.   What portion of the large intestine passes through the pelvic basin? **Sigmoid**

911.   What is the definition of somata? **The soma is the bulbous end of a neuron, containing the cell nucleus. Somata comes from the word Soma meaning the whole body.**

912.   A client 53 years old has a family history of osteoarthritis, what exercise would be helpful for them? **Weight bearing**

913.   Heavy pressure on the mandible is contraindicated. What could result in applying heavy pressure? **Sublimation of jaws.**

914.   Which nerve plexus effects anterior arm biceps and triceps? **Brachial plexes**

915.   In Massaging biceps femoris, what would be the best position of the client? **Prone**

916.   Name the movement of the body toward the midline. **Adduction**

917.   Name some symptoms of muscular dystrophy. **Muscle weakness, apparent lack of coordination and skeletal muscular atrophy.**

918.   Name the crystalized mineral chunks that develop in the urinary tract. **Renal Calculi**
Ca/ Ph

919.   Define Homeostasis? **Homeostasis is a state of balance in the body. The balance is maintained through a series of negative feedback mechanisms.**

920.   What kind of spinal curvature is Scoliosis? **Lateral**

921.   Where is the Zygomatic bone? **Cheek bone**

922.   Define dermatome? **A sensory segment of the skin supplied by a specific nerve root.**

923.   Name the three main categories of Remedial Exercises. **ROM, Stretching and Resistance exercise**

924.   What vitamin is in the eye and can help the eyes? **VITAMIN A**

925.   TRUE OR FALSE. Infection can be a response to stress? **TRUE**

926.   What exercise is used to stretch the biceps femoris?
While standing, place a barbell across the back of your shoulders as you would for squats. Keeping your legs rigid, bend forward at the waist, with head up, until your upper body is parallel with the floor. Reverse the movement to bring your upper body back up.

927.   If the medial side of the foot drops what would this be called? **Pigeon toe**

928.   If you are in a two or three car accident, how would people go about getting the copy of the records of the accident? **At a police station after having filed a report.**

929.   If a client complains of dry eyes and blurry vision, what meridian would be out of balance? **Liver**

930.   What is the zebra striped pattern called? **A dermatome**

931.   What is the name of the stomach's yin/yang relationship to another organ? **Spleen (yin)**

932.   What is Myelin associated with?   **Insulation**

933.   Why would you not apply deep pressure to the cuboidal area? **Brachial artery is in that area**

934.   Where is the governing Vessel? **The governing vessel begins in the pelvic cavity, and ascends along the middle of the spinal column to penetrate the brain**

935.   The Sciatic nerve passes through what two palpable bony structures? **Hip, and the gluteal region and sometimes through the periformis**

936.   Which of the following muscles cross two joints? **Gastrocnemius**

937.   How would you position a client with lordosis?
Put a pillow or towel or even a bolster under the belly to get rid of the exaggeration of the lordotic curve.

938.   Name of fluid would you find in the joints? **Snovial**

939.   What would be the best relief treatment for someone with chronic Rheumatoid arthritis? **Moist heat**

940.   An alcoholic client would show what in Chinese element. **Wood**

941.   What type of stretch would you use for joint pain? **Rhythmic initiation stretch**

942.   Adult blood cells are made from what? Red or yellow marrow? **Red**

943.   Name the connective tissue layer covering the entire muscle? **Epimysium**

944.   Name the only bilateral joint? **Saddle joint (the thumb)**

945.   What is the name that holds the body together? **Fascia**

946.   Homeostasis influences what system? **Endocrine**

947.   In Chinese medicine, what system does Jing influence? **Reproductive system**

948.   Are these two vitamins, B & C, water soluble? **YES**

949.   Name of amino acid that breaks down carbohydrates? **Amylase enzyme**

950.   Does calcium help with clotting? **YES**

951.   What is the action of the masseter muscle and what does it do? **Elevates**

952.   Define is cortisol? _Adernal_ **A hormone for the sympathetic nervous system** _Fight or flight_

953.   What is the middle burner in Chinese medicine? **Digestion**

954.   Name at least three steps to help clients navigate through chronic pain?
        1. **Understand the emotional dimension of chronic pain.**
        2. **Create a safe space for healing.**
        3. **Help client to utilize other healing resources.**

955.   List two functions muscle cells are limited to? **Contraction and relaxation**

956.   Is it true that music affects not only our minds, but the body as a whole? **YES**

957.   Define perfect posture? **A condition where body mass is evenly distributed and balance is easily maintained during standing and locomotion.**

958.   Describe the best way to wash your hands. **Use warm running water using liquid/plane soap for at least 20 seconds, scrubbing palms with your fingernails, rine, and then dry hands with paper towels.**

959.   Name at least five steps that can be taken to safeguard yourself and your business from law suits? **Acceptance, planning, implementation, monitoring and reaction**

960.   Name the technique you would use to help alleviate bronchitis symptoms? **Cupping**

961.   Yes or No. Traditional Thai Massage is shown to reduce pain levels and pain perceptions in patients with non-special low back pain, more than a joint mobilization treatment. **YES**

962.   Name type of therapy for someone who would like to change a movement pattern? **Feldenkrasis**

963.   If you have changed treatment plans several times without a change in outcome, how would you continue? **Refer person to another professional that could possibly help**

964.   Is a chriropractor trained to treat a subluxation? **YES**

965.   What does SOAP describe? **Subjective, Objective, Assessment, Plan**

966.   What muscles are involved in hip hiking? **Quadratus lumborum**

967.   Yes or No. would you use CPR in cardiac arrest? **YES**

968.   What is the color of the 4th chakra, and what is the name of the 4th chakra? **Heart and Green (sometimes pink in other modalities)**

969.   Describe what the manual stretching of muscles and fascia create and promote? **Creates mechanical, bioelectrical and biochemical responses that promote improved vascular and lymphatic circulation, increased oxygenation, removal of body toxins and a more efficient nervous system.**

970.   Name one of the reasons for elevating the lower extremity after a strain in acute stage? **To reduce swelling around the injured area**

971.   In bartering, what should you declare? **100% of the value**

972.   What muscle is involved in a sciatic nerve pain? **Periformis**

973.   Name the muscles usually involved in shin splint? **Longus muscle & tibialis anterior muscle**

974.   If a marathon runner, after their run, has a high fever, their skin is hot, wet and their heart rate is high, what is the runner suffering from? **Heat stroke**

975.   What bony landmark would you locate the kidneys? **12th thoracic**

976.   Yes or No. Can a home based business be deductible for the IRS? **YES**

977.   What is the color for the thyroid chakra? **Sky blue**

978.   What muscles are being used when you are riding a bicycle? **Trunk muscles Quadriceps**

979. Name 4 headache types? **Tension-type, Migraine. Coexisting Migraine, and Tension-type Cluster**

980. What is name of the first vertebra? **Atlas**

981. If you volunteer at a sports event and work as a sports and athletic massage therapist what can be deducted on your federal tax? **Nothing is deductible**

982. When you are implementing tapping techniques, what specific points are being tapped? **Acupuncture points, chakras, or other energy centers**

983. Name reasons why tapping techniques are used? **To move and balance energy in order for the body to heal itself more quickly and effectively.**

984. TRUE OR FALSE. Massage therapists can accept tips but not expect them. **TRUE**

985. What area is the sacrotuberous ligament in and how would you palpatate it? **It is at the lower and back part of the pelvis. You would papatate it softly**

986. TRUE OR FALSE. Massage helps to decrease blood pressure. **TRUE**

987. Name two types of massage that affect both diastolic and systolic blood pressure? **Trigger point and sports massage**   ↑ BP

988. Location where the heart meridian ends? **At the tip of little finger**

989. Location where the lung meridian ends? **Corner of base of the thumb nail**

990. What is Zong Qi? **Chinese Poetry**

991. What is Zhong Qi? **Chinese Calendrics**

992. What is Zhen Qi? **Chinese Herbal Supplement**

993. What is **Wei qi? It is the superficial defense energy.**

994. Name organs associated with the metal element. **Lung/large intestine**

995. Yes or No. Are liver and spleen yin organs? **YES**

996. Name what the upper burner regulates. **Respiration**

997. Name one function of the endocrine system. **It helps in maintaining the nervous system**

SECTION II

1.   Where does spleen meridian begin? **Medial side of big toe**

2.   The heart meridian is associated with what? **The heart is related to the tongue, to which it is connected by the heart muscle. The color and texture of the tongue reflects the condition of the heart. Speech impediments such as stuttering are often caused by dysfunction or imbalance in heart energy.**

3.   What direction does the governing vessel run? **Upward**

4.   An athlete complains of pain in the patella after a sporting event. What area would you massage to best help them? **Quadriceps**

5.   What is the name for scar tissue formation? **Fibrosis**

6.   Name of hormone likely to produce pleasure doing a massage? **Serotonin**

7.   How would you position your client to stretch their Pectoralis major? **Abduct and laterally rotate the arm**

8.   Name the defining characteristics of rheumatoid arthritis? **Joints are red, hot, painful and stiff**

9.   What is a defining characteristic of rheumatoid arthritis? **Chronic and acute systemic inflammation**

10.   In Western anatomical position, where is the distal ulna located? **Medial wrist**

11   Name movement of the radioulnar joint? **Rotation**

12.   TRUE OR FALSE. Contraction of the periformis can trap the sciatic nerve. **TRUE**

13.   What muscle is associated with spasmodic torticollis? **Sternocleidomastoid**

14.   When palpating the insertion of the illiopsoas muscle, what structure should you avoid? **Femoral nerve**

15.   An injury to one part of the body can throw off the entire body balance. What is the name for this? **Compensation**

16.	When you are massaging a client and they begin to have an increase pulse rate and breathing, what could this be a possible sign of? **Anxiety**

17.	Define concentric contraction. **Eccentric contraction involves the development of tension while the muscle is being lengthened i.e. the downward movement of a dumbbell in a biceps curl or when you land on two feet from a jump and <u>bend your knees</u> the quadriceps are lengthening.**

18.	List three suggestions you would give a client who has a Liver imbalance. **Moderate exercise, small amount of sour in diet, rest, cut out sweets, fats and alcohol.**

19.	A client, in the supine position, you have just finished massaging still has retracted shoulders. What would you suggest stretching**? Rhomboids**

20.	TRUE OR FALSE. Shoulder bursitis is contraindicated with friction application. **TRUE**

21.	Name the stage that occurs during the first few days of injury, when there is pain, redness and swelling? **Acute**

22.	If two massage therapists decide to work together, what form would they have to do to keep their taxes separate? **K-1 form**

23.	When would a gift certificate be taxable? **When it is purchased**

24.	TRUE OR FALSE. Osgood-schlatter disease involves the inflammation of the tibial tuberosity. **TRUE**

25.	What would be the best treatment for a client who has chronic constipation and what area would you massage? **Use gliding strokes clockwise on the abdomen-stomach**

26.	When it is time for your client to turn over on the table how would you assist? **You would hold the sheet at the edge farthest from you and have them roll toward you while maintaining privacy for them**

27.	Is massage indicated for all scars? Yes or no. **No It depends on the healing process of the scar tissue**

28.	Name the term for inflammation of the sheath surrounding a tendon? **Tenosynovitis**

29.   Massage may be contraindicated for a client who has_____. **Recent myoardial infarction**

30.   What nerve stems from the brachial plexus? **Radial**

31.   A client shows loss of mobility, tension and elevation in their right shoulder. What could be the possible cause? **Dislocation at the lateral clavicle**   AC Joint

32.   What hormone is secreted by the pyloric antrium? **Gastrin**

33.   Name the three most common causes of back pain?
       Lumbar strain, nerve irritation, spinal stenosis

34.   Describe what Spinal Stenosis is. **The narrowing of the spinal canal.**

35.   When is gastrocnemius in the isometric position? **Standing position**

36.   How do you massage the quadratus lumborum when client feels tired and is in the supine position? **You would have them roll over on their side**

37.   Name the micro nutrient necessary for hemoglobin. **Iron**

38.   Name a possible cause of lordosis? **Back pain - muscular insufficiency of postural muscles**

39.   Name the nutrient that is beneficial for the formation of teeth, bones, the nervous system and aids in sleeping? **Calcium**

40.   Fill in the blank. Neuromuscular therapy focuses on ____ ____ ____ broad categories of health.   **Biochemistry, biomechanical, and psychosocial influences**

41.   Name the muscles of the rotator cuff. SITS muscle group.
       Suprapinatus, infraspinatus, teres minor, and subscapularis

42.   A client says they are fine although they have hypertension, tense jaw, and muscle pains and spasms, etc. what would you do? **Work with them attentively and address symptoms as they come up during your session**

43.   In Ancient Asian techniques, what is the word for transporting energy Qi? **Meridians**

44.   To palpitate the sciatic notch where would you find it? **Medial Gluteus maximus muscle**

45.   Describe how you would work the anterior serratus? **Abduct the arm**

46.   Define neuromuscular therapy. **A comprehensive program of soft tissue manipulation that balances the body's central nervous**

system with the musculoskeletal system. It is used to evaluate the soft tissues in acute injuries, chronic pain or dysfunctional patterns of use.

47.   What would you do first if a client came in with a recent injury with redness, swelling, pain and inflammation? **Apply ice pack**

48.   If you see a client at a social event and ask them what they felt about the massage they had, what code of ethics would this violate? **Private**

49.   What is the most important reason for taking a person's medical history? **So you can discuss contraindications**

50.   What is the first document usually used during an initial session? **Medical History Intake Form**

51.   Of these three conditions: eczema, psoriasis, impetigo, name the one that would be contagious from person to person contact? **Impetigo**

52.   What is the emotion of the liver according to Chinese theory? **Anger**

53.   If someone is having trouble with insomnia, and palpations and forgetfulness, what organ is this coming from? **Heart**

54.   If someone is fearful, restless and had a tendency for edema, which meridian would you focus on? **Kidney**

55.   According to oriental bodywork there are how many major meridians? **12**

56.   What is the concept of/in holistic therapy? **The mind and body cannot be separated**

57.   In laying a client on their side you would do this how? **Place cushion between knees, neck and in front of stomach**

58.   If a woman has gone through menopause what could likely materialize? **Loss of bone matrix density**

59.   In assessing a client with joint pain or immobility, what would be the best way to know what the problem is? **ROM First**

60.   What do you avoid with someone who has diverticulitis or spastic colon? **Stomach** /Abdomen /C|'s

61.   What should you avoid as a practitioner in session? **Wearing perfume, talking too much**

62.   What can yoga do for you? **Strengthens the body and clears the mind**

63.   If you volunteered your services for a charity and you are paid for it, how much do you declare to the IRS? **100%**

64. What is the first and most important thing to do during the intake of a new client? **Listen attentively**

65. TRUE OR FALSE.   Increased fibrin production follows tissue damage. **TRUE**

66. What technique would you use for scar tissue? **FRICTION**

67. According to oriental medicine, what are the three causes of disease? **Internal (emotions), external (the weather and pollution) and germs and diet**

68. Define what neurology is.   **It is a study of nerves**

69. What are two other names for Meridians?   **Channels and pathways; meridians are pathways which life force energy travels**

70. Name some of the benefits of yoga.   **Helps circulation, tones muscles and organs, encourages respiration, promotes energy and vitality**

71. How many major Meridians are there?   **12**

72. In acupressure, what are the gateways to the Meridians? **The pressure points**

73. What are tsubos? **Another name for pressure points; points on the body that connect meridians, and an area of concentrated energy along a meridian**

74. Name the three techniques for stimulating the pressure points and how they all work to restore the equilibrium and strengthen the flow of Qi or Chi. **Toning - dispersing - calming**

75. Define what is 'scope of practice?'   **It is that which defines the practice parameters of a particular profession.**

76. TRUE OR FALSE.   You should use ALL pressure points on people who have High and Low Blood Pressure. **FALSE**

77. TRUE OR FALSE.   You can use ALL pressure points during pregnancy as it helps the unborn child.   **FALSE**

78. When you are working on more than one Meridian in a treatment, is it necessary to open one Meridian at a time? **NO. Do what is most comfortable for you and your patient.**

79. TRUE OR FALSE. Therapeutic Touch is a massage procedure that applies a very deep pressure working around the connective tissue that wraps around the muscles. **FALSE. That would be Rolfing.**

80. Name 3 techniques used in Hatha Yoga. **Breathing & relaxing, various body positions, mental concentration, muscle control**

81.   Why would sports/athletic massage be beneficial after a sporting event?   **It helps to remove toxins stored in the tissues; restores flexibility and mobility, and helps to reduce the chance of injuries.**

82.   Name 4 possible negative effects of exercise in sports/athletic massage. **Strains in connective tissue or in the muscle, an increase of metabolic waste build-up in tissues, spasms that restrict movement, inflammation and analogous fibrosis**

83.   In sports/athletic massage name one reason why deep pressure is used? **used to deactivate trigger points and relieve stress points**

84.   What is the longest, main meridian on the back?
bladder meridian

85.   What type of energy is associated with toning, calming, and dispersing? **TONING is associated with weak energy. When you are toning you use an incense stick which warms the area (the point) and you hold the stick approx. 2cm from the point. Also to tonify at a pressure point, you would hold a stationary pressure for approximately 2 minutes. CALMING - you would use your palm to cover the point for approximately 2 minutes DISPERSING - to disperse energy (Qi) at a pressure point, apply moving pressure with your thumb or fingertip in a circular motion, or *pumping* in and out of the point, for about 2 minutes as this encourages the smooth flow of Qi along the Channels/Meridians.**

86.   What are the four primary tools used in muscular / structural balancing? **deep pressure, passive positioning, precision muscle testing and directional massage**

87.   Where would you find myofascial trigger points? **Located in a tight band of muscle fibers; and found in muscle tissue or associated fascia.**

88.   Name at least 9 benefits of receiving massage therapy.
**improves body alignment
helps in the process of elimination of waste material
improves the oxygen supply to cells
improves relaxation of abdominal and intestinal muscles
helps to relieve tension
helps to relieve sore, stiff joints
helps in the reduction of adhesions, and fibrosis
helps the nervous system
helps to relieve insomnia**

89.   Do most therapists massage by muscle groups?
Yes, however, it is not mandatory but highly suggested.

90.   Name two characteristics of nervous tissue.
       Irritability and conductivity

91.   What is Ayurveda? **It is the ancient healing system of India, and incorporates the triad: body, mind and soul, and consciousness which manifests as earth, air, fire, water and space. Believes illness is an imbalance of body systems that can be revealed by taking the pulse and also by examining the tongue.**

92.   What type of headache is a migraine? **VASCULAR**

93.   In India's Ayurveda healing treatments and applications, what are the three **doshas? Vata, pitta, kapha (sometimes referred to as the tri-doshas)**

94.   , Name the functions of each of the doshas: vata, pitta, and kapha.

       VATA- Bodily air, the subtle energy that governs biological movement/breathing

       PITTA - Bodily heat/energy that governs digestion, absorption, metabolism, body temperature, assimilation, and nutrition

       KAPHA - Bodily stability, maintains body resistance, lubricates the joints, provides moisture to the skin, helps to heal wounds, and supports memory retention

95.   There are pressure points that you should NEVER USE on people who have high or low blood pressure and on people who are pregnant. What are these points and where are they located?

       LI4 - Located on the back of the hand in the web between the index finger and the thumb

       B60 - Located on the outside of the ankle between the ankle bone and the Achilles tendon

       SP6- 4 finger widths above the inside ankle bone, just behind the tibia (never use during pregnancy)

       **K1 - Kidney 1 - you will find this point in the crease in the middle of the ball of the foot, where the color changes from the ball to the sole. Tonify with your elbow to stimulate the kidney Yin and to revive consciousness but
       NEVER use this point if the client has low blood pressure.**

96.   What oils and/or herbs should you never use during pregnancy?
       **Marjoram, basil, marigold, myrrh or rue oils and NEVER USE bayberry, motherwort or
       devil's claw**

97.   Where is governing vessel (GV20) located and when would you never use this point in a treatment or session?

The GV20 is located in the middle of the top of the head between the ears.   You would NEVER USE THIS POINT if the client has high or low blood pressure.

98. Name some of the benefits of using various oils in Ayurveda healing treatments?
Softens skin, reduces stress, calms nervous system, and increases the suppleness of the skin.

99. Name some of the benefits of Aromatherapy?
It can enhance a massage or healing session on the mental, physical and emotional levels and has been used for thousands of years in healing rituals, religious anointing, and for medicinal purposes.

100. What are two inhibitory reflexes utilized in Muscle Energy Technique (MET)? **Reciprocal inhibition and post isometric relaxation (**

101. Pertaining to our body, what would be our first line of defense? **The skin**

102. If you are having a session and the client wants mostly friction, would you use a lot of oils and lubricants for friction techniques? **NO, oil reduces friction**

103. What marma point helps with leg pains and sciatica?
The sprig point

104. What are marma points? **They are referred to as pressure points in Ayurveda healing.**

105. What is another word meaning vascular headaches?
Migraines

106. Sometimes massage therapists encounter clients who have unpleasant body odor. What is the best thing a therapist can do in order to help get the message across to their clients without offending them?
Place a sign throughout their treatment facility that reads: "You must shower or bathe prior to your appointment for health and hygienic reasons."

107. What do the initials ICE and RICE stand for? **ICE: ice, compression, and elevation. RICE: rest, ice, compression and elevation**

108. Yin/Yang is a philosophy about achieving what?
Balance

109. Points near the ends of a meridian are often the most powerful in removing what? **Blocks and in relieving pain along the course of that meridian**

110. These are the seven fundamental lessons in Anma.

    Massage is not just about understanding techniques but polishing techniques as well.

    Do not proclaim yourself as the 'healer.' Establish a rapport with your client.
    Learn to see the body through the hands and not just through the eyes, and always give Anma from Tan Den (the area just beneath the navel where the center of Ki (universal energy) is. It's very important to know how to breathe properly when working on a client.

    Do not use your intuition to make judgments until you've developed enough fundamental skills.

    Imagination is more important than knowledge." Be cautious but don't be afraid.

    Always follow the flow of Tao (the way of nature), do not work against it.

    Center and balance yourself by harmonizing Yin and Yang.

111. Name the endocrine glands and the hormones they secrete.
    testes = testosterone
    parathyroids = parathormone
    corpus luteum in the ovaries = progesterone
    ovarian follicle = estrogens
    thyroid gland = thyroid hormone [thyroxine and triiodothyronine]
    pancreatic islets = insulin and glucagon
    anterior pituitary = secretes 6 hormones: ACTH, TSH, FSH, GH, LH and Lactogenic hormone
    adrenal medulla = epinephrine and norepinephrine posterior pituitary = ADH and oxytocin adrenal cortex = sex hormones, aldosterone and cortisol

112. If a client complained of having shooting pain radiating from the back into the buttock and into the lower extremity along its posterior or lateral aspect, most commonly caused by prolapse of the intervertebral disk, what could this *possibly* be a symptom of? **Sciatica, the inflammation of the sciatica nerve.**

113. What does *Shiatsu* mean? **Finger Pressure. It is a Japanese technique used to treat some illnesses and pain**

114. Boils are primarily associated with what type of bacteria? **Staphylococcus**

115.   In massage of the lower extremity, is the patient usually turned from back-lying to face-lying? **It really depends on whether the patient prefers being massaged on the back first. The patient is not usually turned unless pathologic conditions are such that it seems best to do so.**

116.   If a client has hypertension and complains of being unable to sleep, what treatment would you apply first? **1st, massage the neck and the back followed by total body massage, and a general light effleurage touch.**

117.   A client has had severe arthritis of the whole body for several years and there is a limitation of motion in her left knee; no motion of the patella; and a flexion of deformity of the knee at 145 degrees; what would your treatment be? **You would give her a massage to mobilize the left knee.**

118.   It is necessary for the student of Oriental Medicine to first study the theory of the Meridian System. It is as important as the student of Western Medicine having to first learn, anatomy, physiology, and pathology.
    The 12 regular Meridians (Channels) are listed in the order of vital energy and nutrient flow, with rare exceptions. Please list them.
    1. **Lung (L)**
    2. **Large Intestine (LI)**
    3. **Stomach (St)**
    4. **Spleen (Sp.)**
    5. **Heart (H)**
    6. **Small Intestine (SI)**
    7. **Urinary Bladder (BL)**
    8. **Kidney (K)**
    9. **Pericardium (P)**
    10. **Triple Warmer (TW)**
    11. **Gall Bladder (GB)**
    12. **Liver (Liv)**

119.   Meridians are named according to (1) the organ that is controlled by the energy flow, i.e. lungs, stomach, spleen; (2) the function of the energy, i.e., GV, Regulating Channel (RC), and Motility Channel (MC); and (3) Yin or Yang. In a Yin Meridian, energy mainly flows where? **The location of the Yin Meridians is anterior, therefore it would flow outside.**

120.   Name two therapies that are used to release the flow of energy. **Polarity therapies and Shiatsu**

121.   What are the Yin organs? **Lungs, kidneys, liver, spleen and heart**

122.   In Shiatsu, where is hara located? **In the abdomen**

123.   In Ayurvedic assessment, what are the five methods of acquiring information?
    Academic

**direct perception and inference
questioning
observation
tactile perception**

124.   The Principles of Unwinding is a term that is used in what modality?
Cranial Therapy

125.   Is Russian Medical Massage the same as Swedish Massage? Would the same strokes and pressure be applied to bring about relief of a specific condition? **NO**

126.   What are considered to be the two oldest and most foundational of the healing techniques?   **Anma and Ayurveda**

127.   Are Yin and Yang opposite forces or are they both positive?
Opposite forces

128.   Reiki is based on the principles of Chi. What is another name for Chi? **Energy**

129.   What is the difference between isometric and isotonic?
ISOMETRIC means of equal dimensions, when the force of the contraction is equal to the resistance i.e. when the ends of a contracting muscle are held fixed so that contraction produces increased tension at a constant overall length.

ISOTONIC means having equal tension, denoting the condition when a contracting muscle shortens against a constant load, as when lifting a weight, and when the force of the contraction is different from the resistance, and movement occurs

130.   What is Polarity Therapy based on? **A balanced flow of energy in the body is one of the most important elements for maintaining a healthy body.**

131   Name a benefit of Therapeutic Touch. **It relieves pain and stress and balances the body's energy by applying a light gentle pressure, thereby helping the muscles to contract.**

132.   Name what Chelation Therapy does? **Removes toxins**

133.   Name, in order, the layers of the skin from superficial to deep.
epidermis, dermis, subcutaneous tissue

134.   Define Rolfing.
First of all, Rolfing is an art, philosophy and a science. It is also a form of manual soft tissue therapy and movement education that is devoted to balancing and integrating the body in the field of gravity for the purpose of enhancing overall well being. It uses deep pressure and manipulation of tissues

135.   Define Reiki.
It is an ancient healing technique that originated from Tibet. It uses a very light hand touch on key areas of the body to channel energy to those areas, providing a healing sensation or feeling of energy on those areas.

136.   In oriental modalities the two vessels which travel along the median line on the front and the back are the two most often used for treatment. What are the 2 names and what type of energy is associated with each?
Conception vessel - reservoir of YIN energy
Governing vessel - reservoir of YANG energy

137.   _____ is an acupoint or acupuncture point on the body that can be used for relieving pain, or to produce certain effects to the internal organs and/or to relieve symptoms.   **TSUBO**

138.   What word suggests toward the front of the body? **Anterior**

139.   Name at least five contraindications for Shiatsu or Anma.
Cancer or leukemia; it can spread if you do massage, Fever, If client has suffered from an injury or a trauma within 24 hours, If client has been drinking, and If client has had surgery recently.

140.   What consists of the eight-fold examination in Ayurvedic assessment?
Pulse, tongue, voice, palpation, eyes, form, urine and feces

141.   What massage technique is used more than any other in the western world? **Swedish Massage**

142.   Name three techniques used in Oriental massage practice.
Touching, listening, and asking questions

143.   What is Carpal Tunnel Syndrome and list some of the things that cause this? **Carpal Tunnel Syndrome (CTS) is an entrapment and compression of the median nerve due to postural and structural misalignment. Some of the things that cause CTS are overworking as well as straining muscles of the arms and hands, causing a loss of nerve conductively possibly leading to a loss of muscle strength. Also, constant repetitive movements i.e. playing musical instruments (violins, cello, piano), and court reporters complain of CTS, massaging, typing, writing all day with a pen or pencil while holding improperly.**

144.   Organs receive their autonomic nerve supply primarily from what? **The homolateral part of the nervous system.**

145.   What system belongs to the pharynx? **Respiratory System**

146.   Define Qigong. **Qigong is vital energy of the body. Gong is the skill of exercises for the purpose of improving health and for healing.**

147.   In Ayurveda healing what is another name for energy nerves? **Nadis**

148.   In the West Tsubos are also referred to as: **Trigger points**

149.   Name at least three theories/methods that can be added to enhance the practice of Anma. **Yin and Yang - five lements theory - tsubo**

150.   What is Kei Ketsu? **Tsubo on the meridians directly connected to individual internal organs and supports their functioning**

151.   List at least 11 contraindications in massage.
**Broken skin
lesions covered by a scab/s
person under the influence of alcohol
cysts
blood clots
warts
varicose veins
ulcers
hematoma
herpes simplex
hives**

152.   Would it be a contraindication to massage a person with cancer? **NO. However, this is debatable now. The client should bring information from their physician so you would know. Sometimes it is a contraindication and sometimes is isn't.. Bodyworkers who are not yet trained or up-to-date of the special needs of cancer patients should help the client find someone who has expertise in this type of treatment. Be sure and let cancer patients/clients know how beneficial massage is in the recovering process. Also, Reiki, Polarity or even a light feather touch massage is excellent. We all need to be touched. It is very healing.**

153.   List another name for heel-spur syndrome? **Plantar Fasciitis**

154.   What is Pancha Karma? **It is a term used in Ayurveda Healing from India meaning the purification and rejuvenation of the body, mind and soul.**

155.   In addition to applying pressure on marma points, what else is applied to these points? **Various essential oils**

156.   What marma point sends energy to the colon, reproductive organs and bladder? **It is the *oorvee point***

157.   What does the word Yoga mean? **Union of the body, mind and spirit, sometimes referred to as union with God**

158.   List 3 different types of fungal infections of the skin.
Jock itch, Athlete's foot, Ringworm

159. What is periostal massage? **It is a technique using trigger points that helps eliminate pain and delay development of the degenerative process in the joints, bringing about pathological changes in the periosteum.**

160. Name some of the contributing factors to insomnia? **Stress, anxiety, physical pain and depression.**

161. Name the stroke that is generally used when changing from one stroke to another?   **Effleurage is sometimes referred to as a transition stroke.**

162. The most important thing you can do for your client, in order to maintain a professional relationship, is to be an excellent listener and keep all conversations confidential. Is this true or false? **TRUE**

163. If you were to apply heavy pressure at the back of the knee and were to massage improperly, what nerve would become entrapped? **Peroneal Nerve**

164. What does TMJ stand for? **Temporomandibular Joint**

165. It is extremely important to know the endangerment sites on the body because of the possibility of injuring a client. What are some of these sites and where are they located?
Upper part of the abdomen under the ribs - abdomen

axilla is the armpit where there are many nerves

interior of the ear - notch posterior to the ramus of the mandible

femoral triangle - bordered by the adductor longus muscle

the inguinal ligament, and the sartorius muscle

femoral nerve and femoral artery in the groin

popliteal fossa - posterior aspect of the knee

upper lumbar area - lateral to the spine and inferior to the ribs

ulnar notch of the elbow - referred to as the funny bone

**cubital area of the elbow - anterior bend of the elbow
anterior triangle of the neck - bordered by the trachea**

sternocleidomastoid muscle and the mandible- carotid artery

posterior triangle of the neck - bordered by the clavicle, trapezius muscle, and the sternocleidomastoid muscle

166. Define psychotherapeutic massage. **An alternative method for the treatment of stress utilizing both psychology and massage modalities by a practitioner**

167. It is very important to set boundaries in your own life and in your practice. What is one important thing you should *not* do?
You should never combine your massage therapy with counseling UNLESS you are a registered psychotherapist and massage therapist. Then the alternative (psychotherpeutic massage) would be used if you have the proper credentials, and you and your client have discussed the procedure you would be using.

168. List some of the factors contributing to the formation of our personal values. **Significant relationships with others, nature, spirit and God, meaningful experiences and life changing events.**

169. What muscles attach to the carocoid process? **Biceps, pectoralis minor, coracobrachalis**

170. List the difference between tendinitis and tenosynovitis?
Tendinitis is the inflammation of a tendon. Tenosynovitis is the inflammation of a tendon and surrounding synovial sheath.

171. What is the most *non-invasive* form of bodywork?
Therapeutic Touch

172. What is Anma? **In Japanese it means = The art of Japanese Massage. It refers to the oldest known form of traditional Asian massage and involves stretching, squeezing, massaging and stimulating the body.**

173. When a new client schedules an appointment, it is important for the body worker to have their client fill out an *intake form* in order to assess their client's needs and any unusual conditions. It lets them know what type of services you offer, just as you would complete a form when going to your medical doctor for the first visit. What are some of the questions & info you should have on your intake form?

   **Your credentials -
   boxes where the client can make check marks ( ) to indicate *yes* or *no* to certain questions ---- questions i.e.: What are you wanting to gain from body work sessions? Are you having any problems? Have you recently experienced any major emotional, psychological changes, past traumas? Where do you hold your tension?
   It is important to have a very detailed intake form. Those are just some of the questions you should have on your form.
   Note: Example of Intake Form is in this book.**

174. The word acupuncture combines two Latin words. What are they?
Acus=needle and Punctura=pricking

175. In Oriental Medicine define Gathering Points?
They are points that have a special influence on certain tissues, organs, energy or Blood.

176 Certain points are particularly useful in diagnosis in TCM. What are these points?
Back Transporting Points
Front Collecting Points
Lower-Sea Points
Ah Shi Points

177. What is the definition of a chakra? **A wheel of energy**

178. In Chinese medicine what color is specifically related to the kidneys, lungs, liver, heart, and spleen**?**

kidneys, blue
lungs, white
liver, green
heart, red
spleen, yellow

179. Can blood glucose levels be improved in people with maturity-onset diabetes if they practice yoga? **Yes. The Yoga Biomedical Trust discovered this after doing a randomized controlled trial to study the effects of yoga therapy on diabetes.**

180. What can cause irritation of the sciatic nerve?
Spasms in the piriformis

181. Is it contraindicated to massage a client with encephalitis?
Yes, if in acute stages

182. What is one reason of elevating a limb?   **To relieve pressure**

183. When is the best time to apply sports massage after an athlete has been in a competition? **With 24 hours after the competition**

184. Give another name for a stiff neck? **Torticollis**

185. What is the proper response to a client who reports depression and suicidal thoughts during a session? **Refer them to a mental health practitioner**

186. Name one result of stress. **Decreased immunity**

187. Is the sexual preference of your client considered confidential information? **YES**

188 If a client tells you about sexual abuse, what are some of the things you should say to your client? **I'm sorry you had that happen to you. Do you have a support group that you are going to? You can then suggest that there are several groups that help people who have been sexually abused.**

189.   Jin Shin Do is a form of acupressure that works by releasing what? **Two points simultaneously**

190.   What constitutes an endangerment site? **It is where you would compress blood vessels or nerves**

191.   What accommodation might be made during a session for a client with cystitis? **Frequent bathroom breaks**

192.   When a client does not want to disrobe, what should a massage therapist say? **They will work through the clothing**

193.   Is diaper draping a termed used only for infant massage? **NO**

194.   What is the definition of keloid? **A scar that is thick, ropy in appearance, with excessive tissue build-up. It is also abnormal cell growth.**

195.   What is one of the first things a massage therapist does just before beginning a massage session? **Wash their hands**

196   Client records are confidential except when _____? **By a subpoena or directed by the client**

197.   List four stages of rehabilitation.
**calm spasms
restore flexibility
restore strength
restore endurance**

198.   What is the definition of Kinesiology? **Study of body movement**

199.   If you shake your arm or leg, what is one result you might obtain? **Relaxed muscles**

200.   How much income is reportable to the IRS? **All of it**

201.   Name three consequences of sleep deprivation. **Slow healing processes, fatigue, reduced mental capacity**

202.   What is lordosis? **Exaggerated concave curve of the lumbar spine**

203.   What is one way to ensure a successful massage practice? **Have a diversified clientele**

204.   It is important for the massage therapist to use their body weight when applying certain massage movements. What is considered to be the center of gravity for massage therapists?
The pelvis

205.   Give one reason why most businesses fail? **Under estimate of capital and expenses**

206.   Name leg muscles that are shortened by wearing high heel shoes? **Gastrocnemius and soleus**

207.   What organ is protected by the ribs and sternum? **Heart**

208.   If a client came to you and they recently had major surgery, would you give them a massage? What would be a reason/s why you should be cautious? **Massage can be excellent after surgery BUT DO NOT massage an individual who is on immunosuppressant drugs or who has blood clots. Immunosuppressant drugs are associated with patients who've had cancer surgery or organ transplants. Wait until they are off of their drugs and have, in writing from their physician, permission for massage.**

209.   What are the sensory receptors that are stimulated during a contract/relax exercise? **Propriceptors**

210.   In your first interview with a potential client, should you determine whether they have a condition/s that would be contraindicated for massage? **YES**

211.   What is the meaning of asepsis? **The absence of pathogens**

212.   Name of muscle that is referred to as the bench-press muscle? **The pectoralis major**

213   Define CFS (Chronic Fatigue Syndrome)? **A dysfunction of the immune system. Can be accompanied by swollen nodes, non-restorative sleep, muscle/joint aches and other symptoms.**

214.   Alcoholism is considered, by some, to be a disease. If you were to diagnosis alcoholism list at least four indications.
memory loss
solitary drinking
neglect of personal responsibilities
use it to feel normal

215   Define substance abuse. **Substance abuse is using any substance in dosages or in ways that were not intended to be used by the product or item i.e. food, caffeine, cigarettes, cigars, drugs (prescriptions and illegal ones)**

216.   List the definition and function of the lymphatic system?
The lymphatic system includes the lymph, lymph nodes, lacteals, glands, lymph ducts, and lymphatic. The thymus gland, tonsils, and the spleen are also a part of the lymph system. The function of the lymphatic system is to collect excess tissue fluid invading micro-organisms, damaged cells and protein molecules. Also the lymphoid tissue produces lymphocytes (a white blood cell) that is an important part of the body's immune system.

217. What is the endangerment site in the inguinal nerve area? **Femoral Triangle**

218. What is the endangerment site in the anterior neck? **Carotid artery, internal jugular vein, vagus nerve, +and the lymph nodes**

219. Name the tender spots on muscle tissues that can emit pain to other parts of the body? **Trigger points**

220. You are massaging a client who has varicose veins, would massage be contraindicated distal or medial to the area of the varicose veins? **Distal**

221. Name the bony landmarks where the sciatic nerve passes through the hip? **Ischial tuberosity and the greater trochanter of the femur, bony knob at the top of the leg bone**

222. Where are the landmarks for locating the brachial plexus? **It is the region between the elbow and the shoulder**

223 Give an example of unethical behavior? **Talking about one client's problems to another client**

224. Name the kind of insurance that covers hurting a client during a massage. **Malpractice insurance**

225. List the most important skill during client intake. **Listening**

226. When you are massaging the upper aspect of the pectoralis major, give the name of the endangerment site must you avoid? **Subclavian artery**

227. Define edema? **Retention of interstitial fluid due to protein or electrolyte imbalances, or due to obstruction in the lymphatic or circulatory systems**

228. What muscle pulls the head towards chest? **Sternocleidomastoid**

229 Would massage be contraindicated in edema? **Yes, _if_ edema is the result of protein imbalance due to breakdown in the kidneys or liver. No, _if_ edema is the result of back pressure in the veins due to immobility**

230. Yes or No. If you massage distal to proximal in the lower limbs, could that decrease edema in the lymphatic vessels? **YES**

231. Would massage be contraindicated for a hematoma? **YES**

232. List some of the benefits of aquatic exercising.
**Improves cardiovascular fitness
Increases lean muscle mass
Decreases body fat
Increases Range of Motion in the chest and shoulder area**

Strengthens the back muscles and the shoulder muscles
Helps to reduce stress

233   What is yoga most noted for increasing? **Flexibility**

234.   Specific cross-tissue stokes used in Pfrimmer Deep Muscle Therapy stimulates what? **The circulatory and lymphatic systems by removing toxins; and it also facilitates cell repair, and works for the correction and prevention of serious muscle conditions such as ALS, Multiple Sclerosis, Muscular Dystrophy**

235.   What area would a client report discomfort in if they had diverticulitis? **colon**

236.   What stroke would help in removing waste from the muscles? **The kneading stroke**

237.   How would you recognize varicose veins, and work with varicose veins? **Lumpy skin, purplish color**
Massage proximal to the affected area might be very helpful, especially superficial (barely touching) techniques. Never do a deep massage on small reddish groupings of broken blood vessels that sometimes surround a small protruding vein.

238.   Give an example of an ellipsoid joint. **Wrist**

239.   Do radioulnar joints glide? **No, they rotate.**

240.   What does the Golgi tendon apparatus inhibit? **Muscle contraction**

241.   Does moist heat bring blood to the surface quickly? **YES**

242.   Why would you ask a client to breathe into their abdomen after an emotional release? **It activates the parasympathetic nervous system**

243   What does the term *window period* mean in reference to HIV? **It refers to the time between infection and before antibodies can be detected in the blood**

244.   Is HIV a blood borne pathogen? **YES**

245.   Yes or No. Does HIV die quickly outside of the body? **YES**

246.   Can hepatitis B live outside of the body for up to 3 or more months? **YES**

247.   Does HIV live outside of the body for up to 3 or more months? **NO**

248.   Bells Palsy is related to which cranial nerve? **The facial nerve (the seventh cranial nerve)**

249. If a client is in denial about their pain and frustrations and can't seem to give you accurate feedback about their situation/s, would this be referred to as coping strategies? **YES**

250. What are some of the things that Aromatherapy consists of? **Breathing in or applying essential oils distilled from plants for therapeutic, aesthetic or psychological purposes to help treat conditions and diseases**

251. What is the origin of the short head of the biceps brachii? **The coracoid process**

252. What type of joints are found along the spine? **Gliding**

253. Why do massage therapists not work directly above pubic symphysis? **That is where the bladder is located**

254. Name some benefits of using essential oils. **They are mood balancing and have both uplifting and sedative properties.**

255. Which organ stores bile? **Gallbladder**

256. What bodywork movement is used to break down the adhesion of a scar that is well healed? **Friction**

257. What emotion is associated with the gallbladder? **Anger - you can remember this by saying... "that just galls me."**

258. What emotion is associated with the kidneys? **Fear**

259. What emotion is associated with the heart? **Joy+mental shock**

260. What emotions are associated with the spleen energy and lungs? **Over thinking and worry**

261. What are the bony landmarks used to locate the proximal end of the ulna? **Olecranon process**

262. What does the ulna articulate with? **The head of the radius and humerus above and with the radius below**

263. Is the iliopsoas a flexor of the hip? **YES**

264. What should a massage therapist refrain from wearing while working? **Strong cologne or perfumes**

265. List the 3 classifications of joints in order of greater to least degree of mobility. **synarthrosis, amphiarthrosis, and diarthrosis (SAD... is easier to remember)**

266. Name some contraindications to warm water therapy? **open wounds, fever, bowel incontinence, severe urinary tract problems, extreme high or low blood pressure tracheotomy**

267. Does extension increase or decrease the size of the angle between articulating bones? **Increases**

268. Where would you place the cushion for a client who is lying prone and has lordosis?   **Under the abdomen**

269. Define the definition of vasodilation and would friction or kneading cause vasodilation? **Vasodilation is the widening of the lumen (the space in the interior of a tubular structure such as an artery)of blood vessels.   YES friction and/or kneading could cause local vasodilation**

270. How would you position a pregnant woman during treatment? **Lying on her side**

271. If a client's legs are uneven where else would you find unevenness? **In the shoulders**

272. Name the muscles involved in the flexion of the humerus? **The pectoralis major, anterior deltoid, and the Coracobrachialis**

273. TRUE OR FALSE. Deep effeurage encourages venous and lymphatic flow. **TRUE**

274. How would you massage a client with osteoarthritis? **Light digital pressure along the cervical vertebrae**

275. Define bursa sac and tell where they can be found.
Bursa sac is generally found in connective tissue chiefly about joints and lined with synovial membrane to reduce friction and is found between tendons and bony prominences and other places where there is excessive friction.

276. What is the definition of hematopoiesis?
It is the formation of red blood corpuscles or blood cell formation

277. What flexes the hip and extends the knee?
The quadriceps

278. Is walking recommended in order to prevent osteoporosis? **YES**

279. Is the pubic symphysis a bony landmark on the anterior pelvis girdle? **YES**

280. What is the definition of isotonic solution?
A biological term denoting a solution in which body cells can be bathed without a net flow of water across the semipermeable cell membrane. Also, denoting a solution having the same tonicity as some other solution with which it is compared, such as physiologic salt solution and the blood serum.

281. What is the definition of isotonic contraction?
      Contraction of a muscle, the tension remaining constant; since the contractile force is proportional to the overlap of the filaments and the overlap is varying; the number of active cross bridges must be changing.

282. If a client complains of suffering from constipation, where would the discomfort most likely be? **Abdominal area**

283. In oriental medicine which pulse is used for diagnosis? **Radial pulse**

284. A client who is interested in energy work could be referred to whom? **A reiki practitioner**

285. What are some functions of the integumentary system? **Heat regulation, secretion and excretion, sensation, respiration and protection**

286. What is the function of ligaments? **To stabilize joints**

287. When assessing a range of motion, what are three things that you would check for? **Passive movement, Active, movement, Restrictive movement**

288. Why do massage therapists take client histories? **To determine if there are any contraindications to massage**

289. In Oriental Medicine, Chinese diagnosis is based on many fundamental principles. What are two that reflect the condition of the Internal Organs? **Signs and Symptoms**

290. Oriental medicine takes into account many different signs and symptoms. There is a saying in the Oriental diagnosis: *"Inspect the exterior to examine the interior."* There are four methods traditionally described with four words in the process of diagnosing. What are these? **Another way to remember it is SALT. (See, Ask, Look, and Touch) Asking, Looking, Hearing (include smelling), Feeling**

291. In the method of diagnosis by *asking*, what are some of the things that the doctor and/or therapist should discuss with their client/patient?
The living conditions of the client, when the problem arose, the emotional environment of the client.
Ask questions pertaining to:
fever and/or chills
change in stools and urine
change in sleep patterns
sweating
pain
change in thirst and/or drinking
change in food and/or taste
change in thorax and abdomen area
change in head and body feeling

292. In the method of diagnosis by *looking*, what would some of this include?
Spirit or vitality of the person, complexion, face color, (especially face areas i.e. a bluish color in the center of the forehead which would correspond to the heart); a red tip of the nose denotes spleen deficiency; very short chin indicates the possibility of kidney deficiency. Eyes are very important in the diagnosis.

Different parts of the eyes are related to different organs in the body. An interesting note for diagnosis using the eyes (looking) is if you draw a line horizontally across the center of the eye, the upper part reflects the back and the lower part reflects the chest; also the right eye will reflect lesions on the right side and the left eye lesions on the left side. Breathing patterns, shape of muscles, tongue, channels, ears, mouth, throat, nose, limbs, body, and demeanor are other methods of diagnosis.

293. Define palpation.
Examination with the hands, feeling for organs, masses, or infiltration of a part of the body, liver, pulse beat; feeling, perceiving by the sense of touch.

294. Name 2 definitions of axis?
Vertebral column, the second cervical vertebra

295. What is the atlas? **First cervical vertebrae**

296. How do you stretch the pectoral muscles? **Abduction and lateral rotation**

297. Which stroke encompasses skin rolling? **Kneading**

298. What stroke is defined as a slight trembling of the hand?
Vibration

299.   What could possibly cause a client (while receiving a massage) to have an increase of heart rate and respiration? **The client could have a memory recollection that had caused them to become anxious/fearful, and the heart and respiration increase could be a physiological result of their anxiety.**

300.   Define Reflexology therapy and Neuromuscular therapy. **Neuromuscular therapy relieves tender muscle tissue and compressed nerves that radiate pain to other areas of the body. Reflexology therapy uses certain points on the feet, hands, ankles that correspond to specific organs and tissues in the body and by applying pressure on these points, it can help relieve pain and bring circulation to the corresponding tissues and organs.**

301.   Define CTS, Carpal Tunnel Syndrome. **It is an irritation of the median nerve as it passes under the traverse carpal ligament into the wrist. It causes numbness, weakness and a tingling sensation. Massage practitioners, court reports, and individuals who use the wrist motion frequently are prone to CTS.**

302.   Our food passes through the divisions of the large intestine in what order? **First ascending colon, transverse colon, descending colon, sigmoid colon**

303.   Is a cold application used in the treatment of tendonitis? **YES**

304.   Define fomentation? **Application of moist heat.**

305.   Define homeostasis? **It is the state of equilibrium or balance between opposing pressures in the body with respect to various functions and to the chemical compositions of the fluids and tissues. It is also the process through which such bodily equilibrium is maintained, and it is a modern scientific term that happens to describe quite suitably the flow of Ki (energy) within and among the meridians. The idea behind homeostasis is that dynamic systems (in this case the human body) naturally seek and maintain a condition of overall balance. Whenever an external force is applied to the system, at least one change must occur in the system in order to establish a new condition of balance.**

306.   What's the first thing you would do if someone is having the symptoms of a heart attack? Call 911 and then make them as comfortable as possible by loosening clothing that appears to be tight, then elevate feet 386. The lower free edge of the external oblique is the inguinal ligament. What two bony parts would this ligament be attached to? **Anterior superior iliac spine and pubic tubercle**

307. The lower free edge of the external oblique is the inguinal ligament. What two bony parts would this ligament be attached to? **Anterior superior iliac spine and pubic tubercle.**

308. Define *Resisted Exercise*. **It is the activity of inhibiting muscle contractions initiated by the client.**

309. What 3 things/symptoms can appear when a client has a flare-up of Gout? **Area becomes painful, hot and swollen.**

310. Why is lymphatic massage good for sinusitis? **It drains congestion**

311. What strokes are good for bronchitis? **Tapotment**

312. The purpose of Shiatsu is to effect changes in the flow of energy in a meridian by manipulating the energy vortices called _____? **Tsubos**

313. Four primary principles govern Shiatsu techniques. What are they? **The giver maintains the attitude of an observer. Penetration is perpendicular to the surface of the meridian being treated. Body weight rather than strength is used to allow the hand to penetrate into the meridian that is being worked on. Pressure is applied rhythmically.**

314. Define a herniated disc. **When a disc is herniated, the surrounding annulus fibrosis of an intervertebral disc protrudes and puts pressure on the spinal cord or on nerve roots.**

315. The fluid which flows into lymph capillaries is derived from what? **Blood Plasma**

316. Name one type of bodywork therapy that would help release the flow of energy through the body. **Polarity**

317. Some contraindications exist when using finger pressure to acupuncture points. Where would you avoid using finger pressure? **Directly over contusions, scar tissue or infection, or if the patient has a serious cardiac condition, pregnancy and high or low blood pressure, and children under 7 years of age should not be treated with these techniques.**

318. What is the first symptom that one gets when they are afflicted with osteoarthritis? **Burning, stinging, sharp pain in and around the joints particularly in the hands, knees and hip area**

319. When someone is having an epileptic seizure what is the first thing you would do? **Clear the way of any surrounding objects that might be in the way and make it as comfortable for them as possible**

320. Can massage get rid of stretch marks? **NO**

321. The piriformis is a source of sciatic pain when entrapped by what nerve? **Sciatic nerve**

322. There are several abbreviations that are asked on your exams. RESEARCH THESE.

ROM	= Range of Motion
ANS	= Autonomic Nervous System
CNS	= Central Nervous System
COPD	= Chronic obstructive pulmonary disease
ATP	= ATP, attending physician.
ATP	= autoimmune thrombocytopenic purpura.
ATP	= Adenosine Triphosphate-Molecule that stores energy
PCP	= phencyclidine
AIDS	= acquired immunodeficiency syndrome
CPR	= cardiopulmonary resuscitation
ELISA	= enzyme-linked immunosorbent assay
HIV	= human immunodeficiency virus
HBV	= hepatitis B virus
EDTA	= ethylenediaminetetraacetic acid (edathamil, acid)
TMJ	= temporomandibular joint (dysfunction)
SOAP	= subjective (data), objective (data), assessment, and plan (problem)

323. What are two *possible* signs of AIDS in the early stages? **Night sweats and chronic diarrhea**

324. Is it a good idea to consider, in AIDS prevention, that all body fluids that are wet could possibly be contaminated?   **YES**

325. The following case is being used to illustrate possible choices that can be made using combinations of techniques from three popular systems, namely *Swedish Massage, Shiatsu, and Polarity (information from Beverly Kitss, R.P.T.)* There is also some additional consideration given for this case. One intention in showing a sample case is to indicate how well different methods can integrate with one another. The case also offers pointers for expanding the number of choices and possibilities for practice. It is meant to encourage exploration in the application of methods. The case is not meant to offer stock formulas, as there is no way of knowing how to respond until one is actually present with the client.

CASE: Client: GENERAL FATIGUE

A woman complains of fatigue and irritability after the holiday season. She feels that she cared for everyone's needs except her own, and now she wants to get a relaxing massage.

Possible Session

Swedish Massage: give general relaxing Swedish massage with special attention to areas of tension. Polarity: intersperse Polarity techniques with Swedish massage for stimulating parasympathetic nervous system, thus deepening the state of relaxation. Shiatsu: work feet and hands.

Additional Considerations

Each of our three sample systems has elements that can help bring forth the most relaxed response to the work. In Swedish massage, the tempo and rhythm of stroking and kneading often add to the comfort and relaxation of the patient. In the same way, the Polarity practitioner may use rhythmical oscillations and gentle holding. The Shiatsu practitioner may seek a rhythm harmonizing the pressure and release with the breathing of the receiver. The voice tone of the practitioner may convey certain feelings of warmth and relaxation. There may be a selection of music from which the receiver may choose a piece of special background music. Environmental elements such as heat, lighting, and ventilation should all be checked before starting the session.

Be prepared for the possibility that massage may free the patient to express previously suppressed emotions, for this is a common response and may be as therapeutic as the bodywork itself.

326. Name the four basic steps in a therapeutic procedure that would be specific to a client's complaint. **Assessment, Evaluation, Planning, and Performance**

327. What is the best manipulation for local deep massage of soft tissue? **Deep effleurage**

328. Does Ayruveda (traditional Indian medicine) include yoga practices? **YES**

329. Name of the fascia that holds the nasopharynx open. **Pharyngobasilar fascia**

330. TRUE OR FALSE. Most therapeutic relationships with clients should be Professional. **True. The client feels you can help and are knowledgeable when you act in a professional manner.**

331. Define Sjogren's Syndrome. **It is an autoimmune disease that causes muscle and joint pain and attacks certain glands. Some of the symptoms can include extremely dry eyes, mouth and nose.**

332. Name the style of massage that has the most specific touch and direction of touch. **Reflexology**

333. What structure do you have to be cautious of in the femoral triangle area? **Femoral artery**

334. There are two separate circuits in the process of the blood flowing through the heart. Memorize the below paragraph.
     Vena cava brings blood in from the body to the right atrium and then out through the pulmonary artery to the lungs for oxygen; returns the blood from the lungs via the pulmonary vein to the left atrium out to the body through the aorta.

335. What muscle is affected with the hiatus hernia?
     Stomach - diaphragm area

336. Name a few functions of the skin.
     Barrier to loss of water and electrolytes
     Protection from external agents
     Regulates body temperature
     Regulates blood pressure
     Acts as sense organ for touch, pressure, temperature, and pain
     Maintains body surface integrity by replacing cells and wound healing
     Maintains a buffered protective skin film to protect against microbial and fungal agents
     Participates in production of vitamin D
     Delays hypersensitivity reactions to foreign objects
     Indicates emotion through color change

337. Would Golgi's tendon organ be a sensory end organ? **YES**

338. What is dyspnea?
     Shortness of breath or distress in breathing, usually associated with disease of the heart or lungs, and can occur during intense physical exertion or at high altitude.

339. How does lymph move through the body?
     Flows in the lymphatic vessels through the lymph nodes and is eventually added to the venous blood circulation

340. In massaging the chest muscles (example: the pectoralis minor or major) where would you place the pillows during the massage? **Under the arms so as to relax the chest muscles**

341. How does a therapist determine if their knowledge base of pathology will enable them to safely meet the needs of their current clientele?
     First, it depends on the clientele. According to Ruth Werner, author of *A Massage Therapist's Guide to Pathology*, "If a brand-new therapist is working in a setting where he or she is seeing a lot of clients with complicated health issues," she says, "that person will – I'd like to hope, anyway, find out fairly quickly that more information is necessary.

342. What is the MOST IMPORTANT, MOST PARAMOUNT thing a therapist should be concerned about with their client? **The client's safety.**

343.   What are the five MOST IMPORTANT STEPS therapists can take to further self-education and ensure well-being for themselves and their clients?

(1) Be informed about infectious diseases so you can recognize them in your client and avoid further harm to others visiting the clinic, harm to yourself, and further harm to your client;

(2) join local, national, and international massage organizations;

(3) keep reference books, a medical dictionary, and other resource materials for quick reference about various rare and common disorders

(4) subscribe to journals to be current with progress made in the field of health-related issues; and

(5) read the health section of newspapers so you can stay informed of any local endemics and epidemics.

344.   What is the Rosen Method known for and who developed it?
The ability to treat psychosomatic ailments and it helps clients discover their true selves. Marion Rosen is the founder of the Rosen Method.

345.   Define Hanna Somatic Education.
A system of neuromuscular education which requires the client to recognize, release and reverse chronic pain patterns resulting from injury, stress, repetitive motion, or habituated postures. It is also a hands-on method which teaches how to relieve tension quickly, lengthen and relax muscles, reduce pain, and regain comfort.

346.   What are some of the benefits of teaching parents infant massage? **It can help the parents have a better understanding of how to deal with an Infant who is may have colic or cries a lot, etc.**

347.   Define Scope of Practice.
It defines the parameters of a particular profession.

348.   If you are a practicing bodyworker and you also sell products, this might be considered as what? **Dual roles**

349.   If you are working in an office where there are many therapists and there seems to be several complaints from clients about a therapist what would this be referred to as? **Conflict management**

350.   What are some of the terms of ethics and professionalism?
Supervision, ethics, peer support, laws, morals, professional demeanor, ethical principles, conflict management, listening, code of ethics, disclosure, right of refusal, integrity, listening, delivery information, power differential, standards of practice, delivering information, informed consent, confidentiality,

professional boundaries, sexual misconduct, sexual impropriety, power differential, therapeutic relationship, transference.

351.   Define Gross Income.
       It is the income that is generated by business activities.

352.   Name the part of the body would be affected in case of diverticulitis and what is diverticulitis. **The colon. It is inflammation of small pouches (diverticula) that forms on the wall of the colon**

353.   What is Insertion of iliopsoas muscle**? Lesser trochanter of femur**

354.   When you are lying prone, which of the following muscles on the back range from deep to superficial? **Erector spinae, serratus posterior, rhomboids, levator scapula, latissimus dorsi, trapezius**

355.   TRUE OR FALSE. Scare tissue can benefit from stretching and pulling.
       TRUE

356.   What is the wrong position for a client to be in with posterior varicose veins in lower legs? **Having a bolster in back of knees and lower legs is a "no no"**

357.   TRUE OR FALSE. It is very rare in the Far East and in China for a person to have Asthma.
       TRUE. The development of allergic asthma is directly related to Western life-style. The only time Chinese people get asthma is IF they adopt a Western life-style of eating, etc.

358.   Where does the absorption of the most nutrients and fluids take place?
       Small intestine

359.   Where is the Insertion of the biceps femoris? **Head of fibula**
       What three techniques are used in sports/athletic massage besides those used in Swedish massage?
       **active joint movements
       compression
       cross-fiber friction**

361.   Palpation of the psoas muscle could endanger which structure?
       External iliac vein and artery

362.   What is the meaning of Somatic Practice?
       It is another term for many 'touch' therapies i.e. Swedish Massage.

363.   Would the femoral artery be involved with an endangerment site?
       Yes, it terminates at the popliteal artery

364.   What is torticollis and what part of the body is affected? **Wry neck, muscle contraction on one side of neck causing head to be tilted and twisted to one side.**

365.   Where is the location of the Ileocecal valve? **Between the small and large intestines**

366.   What are three very meaningful questions that confront every therapist?

   A)   What is the first thing I should do with a new client?
   b)   What would be the second thing I should do?
   c)   When have I achieved the goal/s for my client?

367.   What are some of the treatments that can be applied when a person has Ileocecal Valve Syndrome? **Rubbing a reflex area on the front of the shoulder (where the biceps muscle goes through a groove in the humerus) for one minute every other day for two weeks is helpful. It is advisable to go to an excellent D.O. in your area to check for nerve pressure as a possible cause.**

   Note: An open ileocecal valve should NOT always be closed. If you ate an irritating substance, your body in its wisdom may have opened the valve to get the harmful substance through faster. You should go over your dietary history of the past two days before deciding on a treatment.

368.   What are some of the causes of ileocecal valve syndrome?

   Any chronic irritation in the area of the cecum such as an irritated appendix from too much spicy, greasy, or refined food; not enough exercise, water, or any other unhealthful practice that will clog the lymphatic system) can cause spasming of the valve. Foods i.e. alcohol, caffeine, carbonated beverages, chocolate, char-broiled meat; incomplete digestion from not chewing well, eating too frequently, overeating, dysfunction of the stomach or small intestine, etc. can cause dysfunction of the valve.

   Any irritation in the small intestine, strong emotional upset, and overeating a food you are allergic to can cause the valve to become stuck open. Nerve pressure in the upper lumbar spine can cause ileocecal valve syndrome.

   Hyper or hypotonic psoas muscles can contribute to ileocecal valve syndrome too.

369.   List the order of the normal way of walking.
   Heel, lateral surface, then the toes

370.   What is synovitis? **Inflammation of synovial capsule**

371.   What supports the inside of the knee by running vertically from the femur to the tibia and prevents the femur and the joint from collapsing medially toward the other leg?
The medial or tibial collateral ligament

372.   The lateral collateral ligament does the same thing for the outside of the collateral ligament except that its lower end attaches to the head of the _____. **Fibula**

373.   The lateral collateral ligament and the tibial collateral ligament prevent abduction and adduction of the _____. **Knee**

374.   What is another name for the semilunar cartridges? **Menisci**

375.   Of the abductor group of muscles, what three participate with the knee?
the upper fibers of the gluteus maximus
the tensor faciae latae
the gluteus medius

376.   What are the principal flexors of the knee? **The hamstrings**

377.   TRUE OR FALSE. Massage improves immune function in HIV-positive adolescents. **TRUE**

378.   TRUE OR FALSE. Massage eases lower back pain. **TRUE**

379.   There are four horizontal panes to evaluate for physical distortion in Neuromuscular Touch. What are they?
(1) the cranial base
(2) the shoulders
(3) the pelvis
(4) the talus joints in the ankles

380.   What is Zero Balancing?
It is a hands-on method to align body energy with body structure, by correcting imbalances between energy and structure that could possibly lead to loss of vitality, chronic pain and decreased potential for vibrant health.

381.   Can massage help reduce high blood pressure? **YES**

382.   On the anterior medial side of the wrist, which muscle tendons are you palpating? **Flexor carpiulnaris**

383.   No pressure should be used around axillary area because of the _____? **Musculocutaneous nerve**

384. What are the flexors of the humerus?
Pectoralis major (clavicular fibers)
Anterior deltoid
Biceps brachii (short head)
Coracobrachialis

385. What is the best massage stroke to break up area of fibrois (hard tissue build up)? **Friction or deep effleurage**

386. If your client suddenly takes a long deep breath and then starts breathing at a slower rate...why would this happen?
The parasympathetic nervous system has taken over

387. Full rotation in a circular motion of the wrist includes which motion?
Circumduction

388. What is the best manipulation for local deep massage of soft tissue?
Deep effleurage

389. Static pressure on patient who contracts muscle would be what?
Isometric

390. What do shiatsu, acupuncture, and anma therapy have in common?
They use pressure points

391. What system protects the body, excretes waste, and regulates temperature? **Integumentary system**

392. If you are massaging a client and that client wants you to squeeze a pimple or blackhead, what would you tell the client and why should you not do this? **Never squeeze a pimple could cause infection**

393. What is a Yoga Asana? **A pose, i.e. standing, inverted, backward and forward bending.**

394. Which stroke would most effectively address adhesion in tendinous tissue? **Friction**

395. What would describe the effects of fascial adhesions?
Decreased muscle power w/increased chance of injury

396. Which hormone stimulates retention of water by the kidneys?
ADH (antidiuretic hormone)

397. There are two main classifications of glands. Please name the two glands. **Duct glands/exocrine and the ductless glands/endocrine**

398. Which organ is located in the upper right quadrant of the body?
Liver

399. Which organ is located in the upper left area below the ribs? **Spleen**

400. This is a two part question.
    (A) There are five elements that represent the qualities of ki energy. What are they?
    wood, metal, water earth and fire
    (B) Which muscle originates at the sacrum, inserts on the greater trochanter, and is an external rotator of the hip?
    Piriformes

401. Abdominal inhalation requires contraction of which of the following muscles? **Diaphragm**

402. What hydrotherapy modality is used to decrease pain and cellular metabolism? **Ice Pack**

403. The mastoid process is an insertion point for what muscles?
Splenius capitus, the sternocleidomastoid, and longissimus and diagastric

404. The purpose of the pleural fluid surrounding the lungs is to do what?
Lubricate the opposed membrane

405. In which abdominal pelvic quadrant is the sigmoid flexure of the colon located? **Lower left**

406. Digested food stuffs or contents are passed through the large intestine in what order? **Ascending colon, transverse colon: descending colon, sigmoid colon; rectum, anus**

407. True or False? Psoriasis is a skin condition that is scaly, flakes off and is usually red? **TRUE**

408. The muscles of the posterior thigh from lateral to medial are:
Biceps femoris, Semitendinosus, and Semimembranosus (BTM)

409. The parasympathetic system is stimulated by what type of massage stroke? **Long gliding strokes**

410. Name 6 important endrocrine glands.
sex glands (gonads)
pituitary gland
parathyroid glands
thyroid gland
pancreas
adrenal glands

411. Name one type of therapy that focuses on pain relief and explores the soft tissue components of pain. **Muscle energy therapy (assessments)**

412. Which bone is the lateral malleus associated with? **Fibula**

413. What are some distinguishing factors of rheumatoid arthritis?
Fatigue, general discomfort, uneasiness, or ill feeling; (malaise) loss of appetite, low-grade joint pain, joint stiffness and joint swelling, usually symmetrical, may involve wrist pain; or neck pain, limited range of motion, morning stiffness, deformities of hands and feet; round, painless nodules under the skin.

414. The vertebral artery is vulnerable when doing what manipulation?
When massaging just below the mastoid continuing down the neck.

415. What are the muscles that move the mandible?
The movement of Mandible is done by: Lateral pterygoid- moves the mandible medially and forward; Left lateral excursion movement- Right condyle moves forward and medially; Disc- allows the condyle to move freely as long as the shape is maintained

416. How would you treat a client if they had tennis elbow?
Massage the extensor muscles of the forearm and the lateral epicondyle with cross-fiber friction, compression, deep stroking and soothing effleurage.

417. When you are lying prone, which of the following muscles on the back extend from deep to superficial? **Deep layer: intercostals, rotators, multifidus, levatores. Intermediate layer: longissimus, erector spinae, serratus. Superficial layer: Lattissimus dorsi, trapezius, rhomboid**

418. If a client happens to fall just prior to coming to see you for their appointment and they injured their ankle and said they were in pain when they moved it, you noticed no swelling or redness, what would you do in this case or what would you suggest?
Do not work directly on the injury. Suggest they wrap the ankle and go see their doctor.

419. Is it helpful to massage a client who has severe cardiac congestion?
Absolutely not.

420. If a client comes in complaining of pain in their right shoulder from a car accident, what would you first ask the client?
Have you seen a doctor?

421. What structure would be endangered at the ulna humeral area?
The Ulnar nerve

423. Name two tissues that line the surface of the integumentary system?
Epidermis and stratified squamous epithelium

Question: What qualifications does a licensed massage therapist have?

Answer: In New York, specifically, a massage therapist is required to have at least 1000 hours of hands on clinical experience and extensive class room studies of anatomy, physiology, pathology, neurology, myology, and traditional Chinese medicine.
Out side of NY, Inside the US, unfortunately the educational standards are very low. If you are outside of NY, you should look for a therapist that is at least Nationally Certified.

Question: So what makes a "good" massage "good"?

Answer: A "good" massage is usually the result of good communication from both the client and the therapist, trust, sensitivity and strength, as well as solid knowledge of all the body's systems. And of course a comfortable relaxing environment makes it all the better.

Question: What's the difference between spa massage and Therapeutic Massage.

Answer: Typically, though not always, spa massage is done in a general manner, with standard movements that are done the same way on every person. Many spas have strict guide lines that massage therapists must follow, and often they have tight schedules that keep them moving like on a conveyor belt. In Massage Therapy Centers on the other hand, (though not always), your more likely to find therapists who control more of their own schedules and who can perform more 'person specific sessions'. This usually ensures a "better" massage, Why? because each persons needs are so specific, we look at, and access each person as the unique individual they are.

Unlike standardized medicine, the foundation of massage therapy is rooted in caring for each individual. This means that there is no "standard protocol".

Question: How is it even possible that massage is useful for so many different medical conditions?

Answer: In as few words as possible...basically, no matter what disease or symptom your suffering from, there are a few common components; be it pain, muscle aches, gastric problems, immune disorders, heart diseases, and even some cancers, there is most certainly an accumulation of toxicity; cellular oxygen depletion, cellular malnutrition, lymphatic congestion and often a general systemic hormonal, chemical, and even an emotional imbalance that causes suppression of the "normal" healthy dynamic state of our body. You should also know that in fact, stress is a major contributor to all of those conditions. -Massage can cleanse tissue at the cellular level; assist in expelling toxic waist, circulating nutrition to healthy cells, and all the while providing relaxation and an increase of natural endorphin's, that make you feel just great. *(there is a lot of research these days that clearly proves that stress causes genetic break down, this causes premature breakdown and aging. More concerning however, is that current research also points out that genetic mutation brings to life certain types of cancer cells. So in light of that, tension and stress is more deadly then once previously thought.)*

Injury Prevention & Maintenance

Chronic tension may impair performance and result in injury. Stress from every day life, work and habits can create muscle tension patterns that decrease joint mobility and strain adjacent muscle groups. Sports massage will help to align and re-coordinate muscle groups. Stretching and lengthening shortened muscles allows the over stretched muscles the opportunity to readjust - This is passive muscle balancing.

Question: What Should I expect? (I have never had massage before)

Answer: Massage in the US (and abroad in many spa's) is often performed in a dimly lit room. Most of the time the default massage service is European massage (check out *massage definitions* for more info on types). European massage uses lotions, oils or cream, so you will be expected to disrobe. You should always feel comfortable, in control, and at ease. Of course your first massage may make you feel a bit strange if your not use to physical contact, however, the point is that you should never feel judged, out of control, or uneasy. Massage can be strong or soft and may include some active or passive movement. A good therapist will elicit your communication so as to allow you to guide the treatment according to what you are ok with.

NOTE: In the US, as a woman, you should not typically have your breasts massaged, unless it has been deemed necessary and you are under the care of a specifically trained therapist.

However, Americans, be aware, throughout Europe it is common to have your chest massaged, and for good reason.....there is a lot of lymphatic tissue in and around the breast area, so from the stand point of immune functioning and cellular health, breast massage is a good thing. In addition, when breast feeding massage may be especially helpful for relieving engorgement or mastitis

Question: What are the proven benefits of massage therapy?

Answer: The benefits of massage are physical and mental, included but not limited to the following:

* relaxes the whole body
* loosens tight muscles
* relieves tired and aching muscles
* increases flexibility and range of motion
* diminishes chronic pain
* calms the nervous system
* lowers blood pressure
* lowers heart rate
* enhances skin tone
* assists in recovery from injuries and illness
* strengthens the immune system
* reduces tension headaches
* reduces mental stress
* improves concentration
* promotes restful sleep
* aids in mental relaxation

Question: Why do I feel pain in some spots during my massage?

Answer: Pain is very common, and is for the most part it is the result of toxicity in the tissue. Lactic acid, uric acid, and other metabolic waist accumulates in areas that have poor circulation. In order to restore optimal tissue health the sore areas need to be nourished and cleansed with fresh blood and lymph. There are many factors that may be the cause of this pain problem.

Nerve compression from the misalignment of bones, poor posture habits, myofascial strain, tissue toxicity, and poor nutrition are among the most common reasons.

S.O.A.P. Notes

Name: _____   Date: _____

Subjective: A description of the symptoms and complaints discussed by the client (or the referring primary health care provider) that is inscribed using the client's own words. Key words are symptoms, locations, intensity, duration, frequency and onset.

Objective: An account of your observations and results of tests you administer.

Assessment: A record of the changes in the client's condition as a result of treatment.

Plan: A list of recommended action.

Comments: _____
_____
_____
_____
_____

S.O.A.P. Notes

Name: _____ Date: _____

S

O

A

P

Comments: _____
_____
_____
_____
_____

Client Status Report

Name: _____ Date: _____

Please identify current problem areas in your body by drawing the appropriate symbols on the diagrams below.

Key

○ Circle areas where pain exists

⊙ Circle areas with small dots where extreme pain exists

✕ Put an "X" over stiff areas

▒ Draw squiggly lines over areas of numbness or tingling

╫ Mark scars, bruises or wounds

Right   Front   Back   Left

Comments: _____
_____
_____
_____

Massage Therapy Informed Consent

I, _____, (client) understand that massage therapy provided by,

_____, (massage therapist) is intended to enhance relaxation,

reduce pain caused by muscle tension, increase range of motion, improve circulation and offer a

positive experience of touch. Any other intended purposes for massage therapy are specified below:

_____

_____

The general benefits of massage, possible massage contraindications and the treatment procedure

have been explained to me. I understand that massage therapy is not a substitute for medical

treatment or medications, and that it is recommended that I concurrently work with my Primary

Caregiver for any condition I may have. I am aware that the massage therapist does not diagnose

illness or disease, does not prescribe medications, and that spinal manipulations are not part of

massage therapy.

I have informed the massage therapist of all my known physical conditions, medical conditions and

medications, and I will keep the massage therapist updated on any changes. I understand that

there shall be no liability on the practitioner's part due to my forgetting to relay any pertinent

information.

If I experience any pain or discomfort during the session, I will immediately communicate that to the

therapist so the treatment can be adjusted.

I have received a copy of the therapist's policies, I understand them and agree to abide by them.

_____   _____

Client Signature   Date

424. You would encourage a client to stretch_____muscle if they have Kyphosus. **Pectoralis major**

425. This is a statement:
Manual Thermal Diagnosis is a highly effective technique where the therapist uses their hands as tools to feel the changes in surface temperature on each area of the body; from cranium, face and neck, to the thorax, abdomen, pelvis and posterior visceral projections. It is through these changes in temperature that gives the therapist some indications on zones of conflict whereby the therapist can begin palpating the heat-projecting zones.

426. _____ is a modality that does not involve touching the client's body. **Therapeutic Touch**

427. The modality that uses the tongue, pulse, and hara (breathing) in the assessment is called _____. **Ayurvedic**

428. _____ is the organ that is responsible for filtering old, dead red blood cells. **Spleen**

429. Where does lymph return to circulation? **Subclavian vein**

430. These 3 (perimysium, epimysium, and endomysium) form the structure of what? **Muscle fiber**

431. Where is the sciatic nerve located? **Gluteal region, hamstrings and lower leg**

432. When palpating the popliteal fossa, the structures to be aware of are: **tibial nerve, popliteal artery, common peroneal nerve**

433. Tibialis anterior is innervated by _____? **Deep peroneal nerve**

434. _____vessel goes from the heart to the lungs. **Pulmonary**

435. _____ is appropriate for an acute sprain/strain. **Massage**

436. _____is the muscle used during normal, quiet breathing. **The diaphram**

437. _____ _____ muscles are used during forceful inspiration. **External intercostals/serratus posterior superior**

438. What is the correct order from lateral to medial? **biceps femoris, semitendionous, semimembranosus (BTM)**

439. _____is where you would place a pillow while working on pectoralis minor. **Underneath abducted bent elbow, lying supine**

440. _____ would use scented oils and lotions. **Aromatherapy**

441. _____ would be the most appropriate technique that you would apply if a client had spastic colon. **Therapeutic touch/healing touch**

442. Define pes anserinus. **This structure meaning "duck's foot" is created by the convergence of the tendons of the sartorius, gracilis, and semitendinosus attaching to the superior portion of the tibia. Sometimes referred to as 'the bony landmark on the tibia."**

443. What principal are you using when you contract a muscle to increase its flexibility? **PNF Proprioceptive neuromuscular facilitation. Also this principal is sometimes referred to as Isometric Exercises**

444. Working _____ muscle dorisflexes and inverts the foot. **Tibialis Anterior**

445. You are stimulating _____ when you put one hand on the occiput and the other hand on the sacrum. **Cerebrospinal fluid motion or craniosacral motion**

446. Fill in the blanks: _____ muscle is palpated between the iliac _____ and the greater trochanter. **Crest (gluteus medius)**

447. Tennis elbow is best evidenced or indicated by what? **Inflammation and/or some tenderness of the lateral epicondyle**

448. Fill in the blanks. All cartilages in our body have little or no _____ _____ and they tend to heal slowly. **Blood supply**

449. Which bone does the fibia articulate with at the ankle joint? **Talus**

450. If you have been massaging a client and you notice that your client stops breathing, and after you have checked for responsiveness to make sure they are not breathing, what would you do next? **Call 911 immediately**

451. Is crossing friction ever used in Russian Medical Massage? **YES**

452. Should your client, all of a sudden during the massage treatment, tell you they are experiencing some dizziness, complain of some pain down their left arm and some numbness, what is the first thing you would do? **Remain calm, get the client into a comfortable position and call emergency immediately (either 911) OR depending upon your geographical area, the fire department or police dept.**

453. When working with the sternocleidomastoid what artery should be avoided? **Carotid**

454. Define hara breathing. **Hara breathing is when the breaths are directed to the lower abdomen.**

455. When you are working with a client and you begin to notice a very sweet sickening acetone like *odor* emitting from their body, what would you do, and what could be one possible cause for this? **You would suggest they see their physician because it could possibly be a sign of a *diabetic condition*, but remember you are _NEVER TO DIAGNOSE_.**

456. If you are massaging a client and your client suggests to you that they would like for you to relieve them sexually, what are some things you can tell your client? **Remind them the purpose of Massage Therapy and you could also ask your client to leave. If there were problems you should call 911.**

457. What is another word for an unknown cause? **Idiopathic**

458. Red blood cells are formed in what tissue? **Myeloid**

459. Pressure applied to hands and feet is usually done by a _____? **Reflexologist**

460. How often are you to file your Federal Tax Forms, and how often do you pay your estimated Income Tax? **Pay Quarterly and file by April 15th**

461. Why would you want to have Liability Insurance, and please give an example of what this type of insurance would cover? **Liability insurance covers a client falling or becoming injured on your property.**

462. Why should you *not* place attractive throw rugs in your working area? **Client could trip or fall**

463. What kind of stretching of the muscles can cause harm? **When using MET (Muscle Energy Techniques) the therapist should not use ballistic movements against the contractions when they are working with the client in stretching muscles (passive stretching)**

464. Can massage treatments have a positive affect on cellulite? **Yes Massage treatments can have a positive affect on just about everything with the exception of your contraindications.**

465. What position would your head be in if your SCM muscles were contracted bilaterally? **The flexed position**

466.   What type of massage stroke would you use in the mandibular region? **Circular- friction**

467.   Please describe how to recognize a parasympathetic condition. **Watch client's breathing. When it changes and client takes in a deep breath followed by slower quieter breathing, this is the meaning of parasympathetic.**

468.   If a client complains of pain in the hip area and also some numbness down the leg, what could this indicate? **Sciatica and piriformis problems**

469.   You should be careful of what nerve when working on the sartorius? **Femoral**

470.   Joint movement is the strongest when the muscle attachment is near what? **Insertion point**

471.   If your client begins to perspire, this indicates that the _____system is working? **Sympathetic**

472.   Other than Swedish Massage Therapy, what other methodology would involve pressure point therapy at specific points while moving the hands and fingers in a specific direction? **Applied Reflexology**

473.   If you are massaging a client and they start to have an extreme anxiety attack, with profuse sweating and palpitation, what should you do? **Treat it as an emergency**

474.   What is diverticulosis and where would it be located? **Diverticulosis is an inflammation of a sac opening out from a tubular organ or main cavity and it is located in the large intestine**

475.   When massaging the _____region you should be careful NOT to injure the musculocutaneous nerve. **Axillary region.**

476.   The _____ and _____ are considered agonist/antagonist. **Biceps brachii and triceps brachii.**

477.   If a person contracts a muscle and this muscle is pushing against static pressure, what is this considered to be? **Isometric**

478.   One book states Yin is dark|night; cold; inside; while Yang is described as being _____? **light|day| hot| outside**

479.   If a client stops breathing and is unresponsive in a supine position, what do you do? **Call 911, open airway, give breaths, and check pulse   (Standard first aid of course).**

480. What is the anterior tendon that is the midway portion of the wrist near the crease, and what positions provide a full range of motion for the wrist? **Tendon of flexor carpi ulnaris and the positions would be: flexion, extension, pronation and supination**

481. What organ is involved in the production of white blood cells? **The spleen**

482. Name a muscle that spans two points. **Gastrocnemius**

483. In Oriental Bodywork name the Yin organ that corresponds to the Earth aspect of the world. **The spleen**

484. What is the muscle that inverts the foot? **Tibialis anterior**

485. In reflexology, where is the point that corresponds to the neck and head? **Big toe**

486. What is the synergist muscle to the piriformis? **Gluteus maximus**

487. What is the main function of ligaments? **Stabilize joints - connecting bone to bone**

488. Why does injured cartilage take so long to heal? **Because it has little blood supply**

489. Name the joints of the pelvic girdle. **Hip, sacroiliac & pubic symphysis**

490. What is a likely contraindication for massage when massaging a client with diabetes? **Varicosis (Varicos Veins)**

491. What position would you place a client's arm while they are in the supine position, when massaging the serratus anterior? **Place pillows under the arms**

492. In what cavity is the psoas major located? **Abdominal**

493. What is Eastern Anatomical position? **Hands above the head, palms facing forward**

494. Describe how you would give physical support to a client in the supine position who had dowagers hump. **Pillow under head and neck**

495. In the five elements of oriental theory, what organ is yang to the earth? **Stomach**

496. In the five elements of oriental theory, what organ is yin to the fire element? **Heart**

497. What two (2) muscles are antagonistic to each other? **Erector spinae and rectus abdominus**

498. As a massage|body worker, what would be the best response to a new client who refused to fill out the client intake form? **Choose NOT to take that client.**

499. In acupressure the pulse is taken to read the energy fields related to the organs. Where is the site in which the pulse is taken? **The wrist**

500. What group of muscles are involved with the extension of the wrist joint?
extensor carpi radialis longus
extensor carpi radialis brevis
extensor carpi ulnaris
extensor digitorum
extensor digiti minimi
extensor indicis
extensor pollicis longus
extensor pollicis brevis

501. Name a bony landmark for the brachial plexus. **Clavicle**

502. Name the structure that inhibits muscle contractions. **Neurotendinous organs**

503. What kind of neurons pick up information from receptors and send it to the brain and spinal cord? **Sensory**

504. What kind of bodywork is a holistic body-mind psychotherapy which addresses the bio-energetic underpinnings of psycho/emotional distress; produces emotional releases due to the client's blocking of his or her experiences, and expression of life affirming emotions i.e. (anger, joy, fear, etc.)? **Reichian Therapy**

505. What membrane is stimulated in joint mobilization? **Synovial membrane**

506. What kind of joint allows movement in only a single plane? **Hinge joint**

507. What organ of the body helps to regulate body temperature? **Skin**

508. Which artery is used to take a pulse in oriental bodywork? **Radial**

509. Which muscle would you work on if someone complained of patella pain? **Quadriceps**

510. What is the 10th cranial nerve? **Vagus nerve**

511. When massaging near the inguinal ligament what structure would you avoid applying deep pressure to? **Femoral nerve**

512. When applying resistence to the knee while leg extended, what muscle is the primary mover? **Vastus intermedius**

513. If you notice a regular client has a mole that has increased in size, what would be the best choice of action? **Tell the client you noticed it and refer your client to a family physician**

514. What structure should you avoid when palpitating the tissue at the insertion of the biceps femoris? **Common peroneal nerve**

515. What are some of the countries represented in TOUCH FOR HEALTH? **Canada, Mexico, New Zealand, France, Japan, Netherlands, China**

516. What hormone is produced to affect low blood sugar **Insulin**

517. What is the name of the area of concentrated energy in a meridian line? **Acupoint or acupuncture points (small areas of high conductivity) or Tsubos**

518. What organ mostly controls digestion in oriental bodywork? **Stomach**

519. What are the symptoms of anxiety or having an anxiety attack? **Very similar to having a heart attack; panic, quick breathing, can't catch your breath**

520. A client has informed you that they have HIV and you are uncomfortable working with them, what do you do? **Acknowledge it, talk it over and come to a mutual agreement**

521. In what type of bodywork does the practitioner apply static pressure with a low release and a stretch? **Neuro-muscular**

522. How would a massage/bodyworker address a client who has a peptic ulcer? **1st thing to do is ask if they are on any medication; 2nd don't massage around the abdomen area because you don't want to put any pressure near the ulcer, nor heavy pressure on the back opposite the ulcer**

523. What type of massage technique would you use for a person with constipation? **Slight massage in clockwise direction over the intestinal areas**

524. In what layer of the skin are vessels and nerves found? **Dermis**

525. What are the five elements in Traditional Chinese Medicine? **Metal, earth, fire, water and wood**

526. What is affected when a person has a sprain? **Ligaments**

527. In Buddhist thought, what is YIN and YANG? **In Buddhist thought they are the two parts that contrast or exist as opposites of the same phenomenon**

528. If someone was healing from a soft tissue injury why would you apply massage? **To reduce the build up of scar tissue**

529. A runner has just injured his or her ankle. It is swollen, red, hot, and is beginning to turn black and blue. What would it be considered to be? **Hematoma**

530. What effect does massage have on urine output? **Has a tendency to increase the output**

531. What is dermatome? **A segmental skin area enervated by various spinal cord segments; the lateral portion of the somite of an embryo which gives rise to the dermis of the skin; the cutis plate. ALSO it is referred to as instrument for incising the skin or for cutting thin transplants of skin.**

532. What organ is protected by the vertebral column & sternum? **Heart**

533. What is idiopathic? **Cause unknown, no identification for a disease**

534. If you sweat, what system is this? **Excretory system**

535. What is diverticulosis? **Inflammation of the colon, a weakness in the wall of the colon that forms sacs or pouches.**

536. Most of our food is digested where? Small intestine

537 What is an inguinal hernia? **An indirect inguinal hernia in a child is a lump or bulge in the scrotum(boys) or groin(boys or girls) which contains bowel or other abdominal structure which has slipped through a persistent sac from the abdominal cavity. Inguinal hernias occur in 1-2% of boys and about one-tenth that often in girls. Up to 30% of premature infants develop an inguinal hernia. Hernias are most common on the right side but about 30% are on the left side and 10% are on both sides (bilateral). A hydrocele is a collection of fluid in any open part of the same sac and is closely related to inguinal hernia.**

538. Where are the adrenal glands located? **Top of kidneys**

539. Where is the gall bladder located. **Upper right quadrant of the body.**

540. What are purkinje fibers? **The typical muscle fibers lying beneath endocardium of heart which constitute the impulse-conducting system of the heart**

541. What does PSIS stand for? **Posterior superior iliac spine**

542. The apical pulse is located where? **In the fifth intercoastal, 7 to 9 cm to the left of the midline**

543. What are cold applications use for? And to do what? **Reduce swelling**

544. What is the Heimlich maneuver and why is it used?
It consists of inward and upward thrusts on a person's abdomen, between the rib cage and navel, when a person is choking on a piece of food or other object. It hopefully throws the food or lodged object out of the persons mouth.

545. If a client comes to you for a massage and has a stoma, please describe what this is. **It is an opening to a colostomy through which the person empties fecal contents into a bag**

546. What is a prosthesis? **A device such as an artificial limb**

547. What is the normal range for pulse rate in an adult at rest? **60-90 beats per minute**

548. Name the muscles of the back starting from internal to external. **Intercostalis, rhomboids, and trapezius**

549. The extenders of the wrist are on the _____?   **Lateral condole of the humerus**

550. Where is the origin of the wrist Flexors? **Medial condyle of humerus**

551 If your client suddenly stops breathing what should you do? **Open their airway - give two breaths - call 911**

552. Name some reasons applications are used in sports/athletic massage. **Deep pressure is used to relieve stress; cross-fiber friction is used to reduce fibrosis, compression is used to create hyperemia in the muscle tissue, and active joint movements are used in the rehabilitation of various conditions i.e injuries for rehabilitation of neurologic and soft tissue disorders, for Proprioceptive Neuromuscular Facilitation (PNF)**

553. Which quadrant is the liver located in? **Upper right**

554. What would help a client with osteoporosis? **Weight bearing exercises**

555. What is above the pubic and is sensitive? **The bladder**

556. What type of insurance would cover an injury in your office or your property? **Liability**

557. What is the name for the excessive blood in the tissue area (reddened skin) in response to massage therapy. **Hyperemia**

558. What technique in massage would move one layer of tissue over another? **Friction**

559. Rocking and rolling techniques are used in what type of massage? **Trager**

560. What treatment would be used for acute bursitis? **Ice**

561. Shiatsu is associated with what type of pressure? **Finger pressure**

562. Would an ice pack decrease cellular metabolism? **YES**

563. Give one reason why you would have your client fill out a medical history report? **To identify areas of indications and contraindications and other areas of concern prior to giving a massage**

563. What is a secondary effect of using ice massage? **To relieve pain; 1st effect helps to reduce swelling**

564. What are metabolic wastes? **Metabolic wastes are lactic acid and potassium that accumulate in the muscle that stimulates your sensory nerve endings. This build-up of waste by-products combined with the lack of tissue oxygen cause your trigger point pain.**

565. Hot or cold would not be used with a person who has _____. **Neurologic impairment**

566. What would be the best technique to promote lymphatic flow? **Very light effleurage-slow rhythmic movements**

567. If a client seems depressed and discusses the thoughts of committing suicide, or happens to remember a childhood sexual abuse incident, what should you do? **Suggest they schedule an appointment with their physician or a counselor who specializes in those issues.**

568. How much of the money you receive from your clients should you declare on your taxes/IRS? **All**

569. What would the movement be between carpal bones? **Gliding**

570. What technique would you use when beginning a massage session? **Effleurage**

571. Where is the only saddle joint found in the body? **Your thumb**

572. What muscles attach to the coracoid process? **Pectoralis minor, coracobrachalis, and biceps**

573. Moist heat pack is contraindicated for the treatment of what? **Edema**

574. What artery causes the back of the knee to be an endangerment site? **Popliteal artery**

575. _____ churning occurs in the large intestines. **Haustral**

576. Where is the mitral valve located? **It is the valve closing the orifice between the L atrium and the L ventricle of the heart.**

577. What position should the client be in when working the iliotibial band? **On side with upper leg slightly bent and supported over the lower leg**

578. Is impetigo a contagious skin condition? **YES**

579. Tongue and hara diagnosis are used by what type of bodywork? **Shiatsu**

580. What should you avoid when you are doing a powder massage? **Inhaling the powder**

581. How should the client's arm be positioned when you are working the latisimus dorsi? **The client should be in the prone position with their arm raised by side of head**

582. What would you use instead of lotion or oil if your client has greasy skin? **Powder**

583. If a client tells you that she is having a problem and needs to have her chakras balanced, who would you refer her to? **A polarity practitioner**

584. What acts as the stretch receptor? **Golgi tendon organ**

585. Where are the intercostal muscles located? **Between the ribs**

586. Name the condition that biofeedback is mostly used for. **Asthma and stress / anxiety**

587. When you are working under the clavicle what blood vessels should you avoid? **Subclavian**

588. What is a lateral curvature to the spine called? **Scoliosis**

589. Cluster headaches and migraine headaches are called what? **Bilateral and Vascular**

590. Local application of cold produces what? **Vasoconstriction**

591. What are the two most common stances? **Archer and horse stance**

592. Contracting the neck flexors bilaterally would result in what? **Lifting the head while in a supine position**

593. If a client had chickenpox would this be a contraindication for massage? **YES**

594. What exercise is good to increase flexibility and improve relaxation? **Yoga**

595. How would you position your client in order to relax the pectoralis major? **Supine position with pillows under the arms**

596. If a client had twisted their ankle before coming to you for a massage session, and they were limping but said that it was alright, what should you do? **Refer them to their physician**

597. If you are massaging a client and they "get out of hand and become threatening in any manner" what should you do? **Immediately leave your work area and call for professional help, usually 911.**

598. During meditation sometimes the _____system is activated. **Parasympathetic**

599. What is a technique that can assess a weakness in a muscle? **Range of Motion ROM or Touch For Health**

600. Pain that occurs in one area but originates from another area is called _____? **Referred pain**

601.. What is ischemia? **A low oxygen state usually due to obstruction of the arterial blood supply or inadequate blood flow leading to hypoxia in the tissue.**

602. Scar formation is called _____?   **Fibrosis**

603. Where does a strain occur? **In the muscles**

604. What muscle is usually involved in frozen shoulder? **Subscapularis**

605. What organ can be palpated under the right rib? **Liver**

606. What should be avoided at the insertion of the biceps femoris? **Common peroneal nerve**

607. What is the name of the muscle that works against the prime mover? **Antagonist**

608. Where should heavy tapotment be a voided? **Over the chest area and on the back if a person has an ulcer, and below thoracic region.**

609.   Specific joint movements are caused by the _____? **Prime mover**

610.   What are two very harmful foods that are making children & adults "hyper active"?
Sugar, any sugar by-products or foods whose name end in "ose" i.e. maltose, dextrose, etc. And white flour and any foods that have white flour by-products as an ingredient. The movie Meryl Streep starred in on February 16, 1997, on ABC told about a 2 year old boy who was having 90 epileptic seizures a day and was CURED after his DIET was altered. The two foods and by-products were eliminated from his diet. It is important to research alternative ways to get off of drugs that have very harmful side effects, and usually a change in diet with proper exercise can produce what appears to be a miracle.

611.   What is osteoclast and what is it used for?
It is an instrument used to fracture a bone in order to correct a deformity

NOTE: Also, it is any of the large multinucleate cells whose function is to brake down bone to maintain homeostasis and repair the bone.

612.   What is keratin?
A scleroprotein or (hard protein) albuminoid (a simple type of protein) present in hair and in nails

613.   Name 3 contraindications for hydrotherapy.
Lung disease, infectious skin conditions and kidney infection

614.   When the client is in the prone position the soleus muscle is underneath the _____? **Gastrocnemius**

615.   Name an area where you would NOT perform heavy tapotements? **On the chest**

616.   What is a prime mover? **It is responsible for causing a joint action**

617.   What is another name for fat tissue?
Adipose

618.   What muscles are used when you grate your teeth, move your jaw and smile? **Medial and lateral pterygoids**

619.   Name two things cold water application improves.
Stimulates nerves and improves circulation

620.   What part of the body should be raised when massaging the abdominal area? **The knees**

621.   What does compression do? **It pushes muscles against the bones**

622.   Name 9 endangerment sites and their locations

Interior of the ear = notch posterior to the ramus of the mandible

Upper lumbar area = just inferior to the ribs and lateral to the spine
Axilla = Armpit

Popliteal fossa   = posterior aspect of the knee

anterior triangle of the neck = bordered by the mandible, sternocleiodomastoid muscle and the trachea

abdomen = upper area of the abdomen under the ribs

femoral triangle = bordered by the sartorius muscle, the adductor longus muscle and the inguinal ligamentone

cubital area of the elbow = anterior bend of the elbow
posterior triangle of the neck = bordered by the the clavicle

623.   Name the six manipulations/movements that are used in Swedish massage.
Joint movements (passive and active) active resistive/assistive movements
Kneading (petrissage/kneading, fulling, and skin rolling)
Effleurage/gliding (deep, superficial, aura stroking)
Touching (superficial and deep)
Friction (vibration, wringing, circular friction, cross-fiber/transverse) compression, rolling, chucking, and wringing
Percussion (tapping, slapping, cupping, hacking and beating)

624.   How are vigorous manipulations applied? **In a quick rhythm**

625.   Where on the body would you apply light manipulations?
Over the thin tissues i.e. behind knees, around the eyes

626.   Where on the body would you apply heavy manipulations?
On the fleshy parts of the body and for the areas that have thick tissues

627.   The word/s (terminology) of bodywork whether it be traditional methods, Asian, or Eastern the words for energy are what?
Chi, Ki, and Qi and the word energy also.

628.   One should never sleep with their head pointed _____ because it drains energy. _____ and _____ are okay, but _____ is the ideal direction.
South – it drains energy - East and West are okay
North is the best direction for the placement of the head while sleeping.

629.   What is the origin of all forms of Oriental bodywork? **Anmo**

630.   List the Yang Organs.
        Bladder
        Large Intestine
        Stomach
        Small Intestine
        Gallbladder
        San Jiao, also referred to as the 'triple burner' because of the
        involvement of the San Jiao in metabolism, burner meaning
        'metaboliser.

631.   List the Yin Organs.
        Liver
        Pericardium
        Heart
        Lung
        Spleen
        Kidney

632.   What are the qualities of the three doshas?
        Vata is responsible for all movement in the body
        Pitta is responsible for all metabolisms in the body
        Kapha is responsible for all structure & lubrication in the body

633.   What are Srotas? **Srotas, meaning channels or pores, are present**
        throughout the visible body as well as at the "invisible" or
        subtle level of the cells, molecules, atoms, and subatomic
        strata. It is through these channels that nutrients and other
        substances are transported in and out of our physiologies. It is
        also through these channels that information and intelligence
        spontaneously flow.

634.   What are Marmas? **Marmas are conjunction points of**
        consciousness in the body. There most common application is in
        Ayurvedic massage. There are 108 major marmas in the body.

635.   List the meridians in the body.
        Heart
        Small Intestine
        Stomach
        Spleen
        Bladder
        Kidney
        Pericardium
        Triple Warmer
        Gall Bladder
        Liver
        Lung
        Larger intestine
        Central or Conception vessel
        Governing vessel

Yin
Yang
The Five Elements

636.   Define Cun. **It is a unit of measure to locate an acupuncture point either on a human or an animal.**

637.   Define meridians. **Channels of energy that flow up and down the body with relationship to the internal organs.**

638.   What is cryotherapy? **Application of ice**

639.   What is orthobionomy and who were two individuals who formalized and modified this modality?

   Ortho-Bionomy® is a gentle yet very effective technique that eases stress and promotes relaxation. Working with the body's structure Ortho-Bionomy facilitates the therapeutic process and promotes natural body alignment, balance and pain relief. Ortho-Bionomy uses gentle movements, comfortable positioning and compression to restore balance. There were two doctors who played a role in this modality. They are Dr. Pauls and Dr. Jones.

641.   What does the glenohumeral joint consist of? **Humerus and scapula**

642.   Describe what an 'effort' is? **It is a force applied to a lever to overcome resistance.**

643   If you have been riding a bicycle for a very long distance, name the nerve that is sometimes irritated? **Pudendal**

SECTION III
WORDS TO BECOME FAMILIAR WITH

Acupuncture points
Nadi
Kundalini
Sushumna
Brahmand
Shiatsu
Prana
Dharma
Ayurveda
Cun
Moxibustion
Kyo
Jitsu
Tsubos
Client and Practitioner agreement and policy statements
Career
Reciprocity
Deduction
Taxes
Ledger
Budget
Overhead
Income
Gross Income
Net Income
Expense
DBA – Doing Business As….
Corporation
Sole proprietor
Partnership
LLC
Mission Statement
Burnout
Law and Legislation
Touch Techniques
Diversity and Touch
Gender Issues
Erotic and/or sexual touching
Advertising
Business Cards
Location of business
Independent Contractor
Licenses
Records
Paper Trails

Bookkeeping Procedures
Third Party Reimbursement
Word of Mouth
Brochures
Dissociative Behavior
PTS Post Traumatic Stress
Mobility
Prenatal
Post Natal
Credentials
Banking Procedures for Business
Receiving Cash for your services
Start Up Costs
Interview Questions and Procedures
Intake Form
Terminal Illness
Things pertaining to physically challenged i.e. Visual, hearing, mobility, size
Things pertaining to psychologically challenged i.e. trauma, psych disorders
Things pertaining to wellness i.e. coping, nutrition, sleep, behavior, etc.
Post Event – usually pertains to athletes
Pre Event – same as above
Restorative Massages
Rehabilitation massages
Remedial Massages
Recovery Massages
Trigger Point Therapy- Learn the major trigger points and methods of treatment
Ambulatory
Phantom pain
Visceral
Viral
Idiopathic
Congenital
Anaplasia
Malignant
Somatic
Bacterial
Symptom

Descriptions of Various Therapies [1]

Acupuncture - is a means of contacting the electrical centers of the body and influencing the flow of energy (chi) to bring about a balance between positive and negative (yin-yang) forces. The energy or chi travels throughout the body by means of pathways called meridians. Needles are used to stimulate various points along these meridians. Massage and cauterization may also be used as stimulants.

Alexander Method - Fredrich Alexander believed that many illnesses can be traced to the way we use our bodies. Unconsciously, we have picked up poor body habits early in childhood from those around us. Also, stressful, urban life contributes to misuse of the body. The Alexander Method consists of techniques for unlearning the old habits so that the natural body can take over.

Applied Kiniesiology - is a system which is used by a primary health care provider to analyze our structural, chemical, and mental aspects of health. It uses muscle testing, postural analysis, gait analysis, along with other standard methods of diagnosis to assess and treat functional health problems as opposed to pathological health problems. Included in the Applied Kiniesiology approach are specific joint manipulations, various myofacial therapies, cranial techniques, meridian therapy, clinical nutrition, dietary management, and various reflex procedures.

Aromatherapy - is the enhancement of body, mind, and spirit with aromatic, botanical essential oils. The essential oil of each plant is its life force containing both medicinal and aromatic characteristics, and it remains potent and stable when properly extracted from the plant. These oils are obtained from the various parts of plants: leaves, flowers, bark, stems, berries, fruits, and roots. The oils provide tremendous healing and balancing properties when used according to proper guidelines. Most often used in baths, massages, and inhalations, they are readily absorbed through the skin and, when inhaled, they affect the brain and its release of neuro-chemicals. Depending on the essential oil used, aromatherapy can help you relax, enjoy, rejuvenate, increase mental alertness, and much, much more.

Aura and Color Healing - The electromagnetic field which surrounds the body is the aura. It is said that illness begins in the aura long before it reaches the physical body. A "sensitive" healer is able to diagnose by means of his/her visual perception of the aura.

The affected organ or area shows up dark or grayish on the multi-colored aura. A color healer will apply remedial colors where a color deficiency exists or contrasting colors where there is an excess. Colors are applied actually or by means of visualization.

Ayurvedic Healing - is an ancient Indian science of life whose purpose is to allow one to understand his/her constitutional makeup and choose the diet and living condition best suited to his/her particular needs. This system uses only natural means of treatment and prevention of disease through herbs, oils, minerals, massage, heat, water, yoga, meditation, elimination therapy, diet, and life style management.

Bach Flower Remedies - Edward Bach believed that physical disease was caused by moods such as worry, fear, shock, etc. Bach used flower; bud, and twig essences in order to treat moods and thus disease. Specific flowers are suggested for balancing specific mind states.

Bates Lye System - This is a system for strengthening and developing the eyes. All eyesight disorders are seen as a result of strain that can be mental, emotional, or physical. In a relaxed state, the eye sees perfectly. Bad eyesight comes from chronic tension. Various exercises and techniques are practiced.

Bioenergetics - is a bodywork approach based on the premise that the body contains and expresses everything that happens to the individual. The body reflects who I am and how I operate in the world. Bioenergetic exercises are designed to open blocked or tensed areas of the body. As the body opens, so do the emotions and attitudes.

Biofeedback - Technological devices monitor the unconscious processes and feedback this information to the conscious mind. Thus the conscious mind learns to control the unconscious, to direct healing energy, and to restore balance.

Biorhythms - Your physical, mental, and emotional cycles all have a special and individual relationship to each other. By plotting and charting the physical 23-day cycle, the creative and emotional 28.day cycle, and the intellectual 33-day cycle, you can take full advantage of the individual energy patterns in daily life.

Chakra - is a Sand script word meaning wheel. The chakras are force centers or vortices through which energy flows from one of man's bodies to another. Disciplines do not agree as to how many chakras exist: some say 5, others say 7, and still others say 10.However many, all these wheels are perpetually rotating, receiving, and directing energies. There are corresponding areas on the physical body for each chakra: at the base of the spine, over the spleen, at the navel or solar plexus, over the heart, at the front of the throat, just above the space between the eyebrows, and on the top of the head.

Chiropractic - is the study of problems of health and disease from a structural point of view. Special consideration is given to spinal mechanics and neurological relations- disease may he caused or aggravated by disturbances of the nervous system: disturbances of the nervous system may have caused derangements of the muscular, skeletal structures. Chiropractic does not use drugs, medicines, or operative surgery in its treatment.

Colon Therapy - is sometimes referred to as colon irrigation or colonics or colon therapy. These are all names for the process which uses water for inner cleansing. Colonics are the gentle infusion of water into the colon-water goes in fecal matter is flushed out (the water is normally body temperature). A patient should always investigate the sterilization of instruments used by their colonic practitioner. The use of disposable rectal nozzles is obviously the most sterile. To a professional, health and safety must be of primary importance.

Cranio-Sacral Therapy - is a gentle method of evaluating and enhancing the function of the craniosacral system, a physiological fluid circulatory system that surrounds and protects the brain and spinal cord. This non-invasive manual therapy enhances the body's natural healing processes. It has been proven effective in treating a wide range of medical problems associated with pain and dysfunction.

Feldenkrais - Dr. Moshe Feldenkrais sees movement and the organization of movement as a key to understanding the relation of life style, self organization, and health. But even more important, Dr. Feldenkrais sees the reorganization of movement as a pathway to the kind of self reorganization resulting in the ability to lead a more healthy, stress adaptable, and efficient life. To this end he has spent the last forty years of his life developing a teaching based on awareness to help people learn to use themselves in less destructive and healthier ways.

Gestalt - seems to be a way of living rather than a therapy. Gestalt focuses on moment-to-moment awareness of the individual in all his/her detail and complexity. Gestalt is first a philosophy, a way of being, and then superimposed are ways of applying this knowledge so others can benefit from it.

Grof's Holotropic Breath Work - is a powerful technique of self-exploration and healing, based on and combining insights from modern consciousness research, depth psychology, and various spiritual practices. This approach is based on the mobilization of the spontaneous healing potential of the psyche in non-ordinary states of consciousness which are induced by breathing and evocative music. Holotropic Breath work mediates access to all levels of human experience including unfinished issues from postnatal biography, sequences of psychological death and rebirth, and the entire spectrum of transpersonal phenomena.

Homeopathy - was first formulated in the early 1800's by Dr. Samuel Hahnemann. Homeopathy's basic premise is that a substance which, in overdose, causes symptoms in a healthy person, will cure these same symptoms in a sick person when given in infinitesimal doses. However, before a homeopathist prescribes, the entire person, as well as the symptoms, are researched quite carefully.

Hypnotherapy - uses hypnosis as a psychotherapeutic tool. The altered state that occurs under hypnosis has been compared to a state of deep meditation or transcendence, in which the innate recuperative abilities of the psyche are allowed to flow more freely. The client can achieve greater clarity regarding his/her own wants and needs, explore other events or periods of life requiring resolution, or generally develop a more positive attitude. Hypnotherapy has also been particularly effective with stress disorders and various addictions.

Iridology- A means of revealing the pathological and functional disturbances in the body by reading the markings in the iris and surrounding areas of the eye. The iris is the most complex tissue of the body meeting the outside world. It is an extension of the brain, being endowed with hundreds of nerve endings, microscopic blood vessels, muscle and other tissues. Location of disease, its history and progression, and even clues to the cure, can be read in the eyes.

Kundalini Yoga - is the releasing of the coiled serpentine energy which resides at the base of the spine. This release is brought about by practicing a combination of postures, breathing patterns, mudras (hand or finger positions), and meditation techniques.

Macrobiotics - was begun over 70 years ago and popularized by Dr. George Oshawa who broadened the system to embrace the whole individual. He treated illness with natural foods and used no medicines. The diet is based on the yin-yang principle; all foods fall into one or the other category. If foods are properly chosen and combined, bodily balance can be restored in those who have fallen ill. Brown rice is said to he perfectly balanced between yin and yang. Proper or balanced diet is said to eliminate illness, fatigue, and to stimulate creative life.

Magnetic Healing - The healer attracts and transmits energy necessary to counteract the patient's disease. At the same time, the healer draws the energy associated with the illness from the patient. That energy is absorbed by the healer and later either transformed or shed. Most practitioners have favorite ways of ridding themselves of energy associated with sickness.

Mitzvah Technique - is a reeducation and functional integration discipline, developed by M. Cohen-Nehemia, formerly of Israel, founder of The Canadian Mitzvah Technique Center and Training School. The technique is based upon a self-organizing ability, which is both preventative and remedial. Cohen's research and teaching demonstrates the body's self-organizing ability (seen clearly in young children) as an upward rippling motion of the spine with each movement of the pelvis-bringing with it a dynamic relationship between the pelvis, spine, and head, promoting spinal integrity. Habitual body misuse, occupation or accident, interferes with the pelvis, spine, and head dynamics, causing postural changes (eg., the chin pokes, the head retracts, the back hunches, the chest caves, and the body twists), resulting in diverse pains (back, hip, neck, shoulder, sciatica, and breathing difficulties). The Mitzvah Technique aims at restoring the body's self-organizing ability.

Massage - There are many different kinds of massage, but all of them touch the self or another in varying intensities of pressure. The contact can be used in a variety of ways: to increase the circulation by dilating the blood vessels, to stimulate the lymph circulation which aids in the elimination of wastes and toxic debris, to increase the blood supply and nutrition to the muscles and tissues, to improve muscle tone, etc.

Naturopathy - is a form of primary health care that has been practiced in North America since the turn of the century. Naturopaths recognize the inherent ability of the body to heal itself and act to identify and remove obstacles to its recovery. The naturopathic practitioner seeks to detect and eliminate the underlying causes of illness, rather than to merely suppress the symptoms. Naturopathic practitioners treat the whole individual, taking into account each patient's physical and mental health, genetic predispositions, and environmental influences. They also emphasize a preventive approach to disease and encourage self responsibility for health care. The Naturopathic approach can prevent minor illnesses from developing into more serious or chronic degenerative diseases. Patients are taught the principles by which to live a healthy life. The modern naturopathic practitioner provides a comprehensive range of diagnostics, treatments and therapies, and if necessary, referral to the appropriate specialist.

Network Chiropractic - is a network of many methods utilized in chiropractic today. Its practitioners view the spine as a powerful "switchboard of consciousness." In this approach, specific sequencing of both traditional light touch and structural chiropractic techniques are utilized. Rather than naming and treating symptoms and diseases, the practitioner locates subluxation at the spinal level and adjusts them. This frees mechanical tensions from the spinal system, empowering the innate intelligence to more fully express itself.

Neurolinguistic Programming (NLP) - is a comprehensive approach to developing more effective communication skills. It studies the different sensory levels through which we absorb information and how we organize, create, are motivated by, and make decisions, according to our own individual patterns of perception. Therapeutically, NLP has been used in work with phobias, learning disabilities, addictive behavior, and the development of new talents and more desirable, constructive behavioral patterns.

Polarity Therapy - This system views the body as a balanced electromagnetic field. The right side is charged with positive energy and the left side with negative energy. Too much positivity is associated with heat, inflammation, irritation, and swelling. Too much negative energy is associated with tension, spasm, and poor circulation. The aim of the therapy is to balance the energies in the body.

Posture Perfect - is a program developed by Robert Toporek, an advanced certified Rolf practitioner. Using the techniques and principals of Rolfing, Robert has taken the work of Ida Rolf beyond the traditional practice. The Posture Perfect program enables a person to undo postural patterns developed through a life of stress, trauma, and tension. In addition, this program addresses the patterns you have inherited and developed from birth. Posture Perfect gives you unimagined freedom in your body and life. By gently stretching muscle and connective tissue, tension and trauma are removed from your body. Through education you are given the tools to live into your new posture. People often report feeling looser, lighter, and being more productive with much less effort.

Rebirthing- is a safe and powerful breathing process that releases tension from the body, freeing it, so that we may live to our highest vision and unlimited potential. The breath is the ultimate healer. It is the umbilical cord to the divine. By using a variety of smoothly connected breaths, energy which may be called Prana, Chi or Ki, or life force, is taken into the body dissolving
and washing away anything that is contrary to life. When this takes place we become aware of our blocks and what has been holding us back; an inner cleansing occurs.

Reiki - is an ancient form of healing traced back to Tibet thousands of years ago. This technique was rediscovered in the 19th century by Dr. Mikao Usui, a Japanese Christian educator. Reiki is a hands.on, non-invasive healing technique. The word "reiki" is a combination of Japanese symbols when combined, present the concept of "Universal life-force energy." The client participates in their own healing. The reiki practitioner is a channel and a clear vessel through which the healing energy flows. Reiki energy allows us to heal ourselves spiritually, emotionally, mentally, and physically.

Reflexology - Strong massage of the feet at certain reflex points which correspond to the various areas and organs of the body. Reflexology points are different from acupuncture points. Foot treatments are said to dissolve the hardened toxins which accumulate in the body in the form of tiny crystals. Once the crystals are released into the bloodstream, they are eliminated naturally by the body. Circulation is increased and organs and glands are stimulated.

Rolfing - is an original and scientifically validated system of body restructuring & movement education. It releases the body's segments-- legs, torso, arms, etc- from lifelong patterns of tension and bracing, and permits gravity to realign them. By doing so, it balances the body. Because the body is better-balanced after Rolfing, it expends less of its vital energies against gravity. This biological energy-efficiency is often experienced as a higher level of alertness and vitality. Movement becomes easier and overall personal functioning tends to improve.

St. John Method of Neuromuscular Therapy - is a comprehensive system of soft-tissue manipulation techniques that balance the central nervous system (brain, spinal cord, and nerves) with the musculo-skeletal system. Therapists use these soft tissue correction techniques to restore proper functioning to muscles, which helps relieve pain and dysfunction.

Shiatsu Japanese- Finger pressure is applied to acupuncture meridian points by a practitioner. The pressure stimulates and balances the energy flowing through the body. A total body treatment employing the application of appropriate pressure to the meridians of the body according to the Oriental medical model. Pressure is applied mainly with the thumbs, but also with palms, elbows, and knees, to stimulate the flow of Qi (Chi or Ki), or energy, thereby promoting the self healing abilities of the body. A goal of Shiatsu is to facilitate a calming response and to maintain or restore physical function and/or relieve pain.

T'ai Chi - is a Chinese Taoist martial art form of meditation in movement, combining mental concentration, coordinated breathing, and a series of slow, graceful body movements. T'ai Chi may be practiced for meditative and health purposes or, with increased speed, the movements may be used for self-defense. The practitioner allows the body weight or center of gravity to sink into the abdomen and feet; this relaxes and deepens the breathing, quiets the mind and, in turn, regulates the heartbeat digestion, and various other muscular neurological, glandular and organic functions.

Trager Approach - is based on a simple concept: much discomfort, tension, stiffness and fatigue can be released by imparting to the nervous system a different set of signals. In this case, motion in the muscles and joints is used to communicate the sensations of lightness, ease, freedom, pleasure and aliveness. To experience these feelings in moving and being is to learn how to replace restriction with freedom in moving and being. These positive pleasurings are imparted (1) via gentle, non-invasive bodywork (psychophysical integration), and (2) through the teaching of simple, mindful movement explorations (Mentastics) which the client uses to generate these sensations on his/her own.

Unergi: Unity and Energy. A Holistic Therapy Method developed by Ute Arnold. It interweaves body awareness, movement, safe and healing touch, talk, dialoguing, inner listening, visualization and meditation, dream work, remembering, creative expression (especially visual art, music, and dance), ritual, accessing the woundedness, wisdom, playfulness of one's inner child, and attunement to nature; along with healing forms derived from Gestalt Therapy, Feldenkrais Movements, the Alexander Technique, and Rubenfeld Synergy.

Yoga - A spiritual technology or system whereby the practitioner can directly experience interior reality. The word yoga is derived from the Sand script, meaning to bind, to join, attach or yoke, to direct and concentrate attention on, to use and apply. Yoga techniques and postures often assist in adding flexibility to the body while focusing the mind. Click here for more Information on Yoga and Life Enrichment Network Yoga Instructors

Vitamins, Minerals, & Herbs

People report that vitamins, minerals, & herbs can be powerful and effective in improving health. Since they can interact in different ways with medications and since each person's needs differ, please check with your physician and/or primary care provider before taking. Also, make certain you follow your physician's or the company's dosage instructions.

Vit. A - Helps to maintain good vision, prevents night blindness, and dryness of the eyes; aids in growth, repair, and maintenance of body tissues. Helps form strong bones, teeth, and gum It is essential for pregnant or lactating women; it occurs in significant amounts in fish-liver oils, animal liver, eggs, and whole milk.

Beta-Carotene - Known to strengthen the immune system. Maintains healthy skin and eyes, prevents night blindness, and protects skin from ultra-violet rays.

Vit. B (Complex) - A family of essential water-soluble vitamins which complement each other. Helps to combat negative effects of caffeine, nicotine, alcohol, antibiotics, fats, and sugar. Relieves effects of stress, strenuous exercise or improper diet.

Vit. B1 (Thiamine) - Important for metabolizing carbohydrates into energy and for normal function of the nervous system. Help in poor muscular and circulatory performance. Thiamine needs are increased during illness, stress, after surgery. Found in lean pork, beans, dried peas and nuts, liver, meats, milk, eggs.

Vit. B2 (Riboflavin) - Required for vision, growth, absorption of iron. Essential for healthy skin, nails, hair, eyes, as well as the formation of antibodies. Can be destroyed by light, heat, and air; it is often deficient in the diet. If you have cracks in the corner of your mouth and have light sensitivity of the eyes, you may be deficient in this vitamin. Found in beef, chicken, liver, salmon, nuts, beans and leafy greens.

Vit. B3 (Niacinamide) - Involved in hundreds of biochemical reactions in the body. Essential for normal body balance and the health of our nervous system.

Vit. B5 (Pantothenic Acid) - Essential for the synthesis of cholesterol and fatty acids and maintaining a healthy digestive tract. Important to normal immune system function. Deficiencies produce biochemical defects, retarded growth rate in animals, cramping and impairment of motor coordination. Found in the honey bee's "royal jelly."

Vit. B6 (Pyridoxine HCl) - Required for processing fats, carbohydrates and protein, utilizing linoleic acid an the production of antibodies and red blood cells. Lack of it may result in anemia, fatigue and hyper irritabilit. Found in bananas and raw steak.

Vit. B12 (Cyanoco Balamin) - Aids the normal synthesis of red blood cells and proper utilization of fats, carbohydrates, and protein. Lack of this vitamin may result in red and sore tongue, anemia and general fatigue,. B12 is absent from most fruits, vegetables, grains. Found in meats, animal products, tempeh, and other vegetarian sources.

Vit. B15 - Helps increase oxygen supply to active tissue. Beneficial for those involved in strenuous exercise as it may prevent lactic acid build up.

Choline - Essential for the health of kidneys, liver, and arteries. A fat emulsifying agent which aids in the burning of intermuscular fat. Essential for normal nerve transmission, gall bladder regulation, lecithin formulation.

Inositol - Essential for the growth and color of hair, healthy intestinal activity, control of blood cholesterol, health of bone marrow and eye membranes.

PABA (Para Amino Benzoic acid) - A growth factor, PABA helps utilize protein and is important in the maintenance of healthy skin and hair.

Biotin - Aids in metabolizing carbohydrates and fats into energy. As a growth-promoting factor, it is important for the development of healthy hair, skin, and muscles. Found in liver, oysters, eggs, beans, peanuts.

Folic Acid - Essential in synthesizing DNA and RNA. Also important for the formation of red blood cells, protein metabolism, reproduction and growth. Lack of it may cause gastrointestinal distress. Found in spinach.

Vit. C - Essential in the formation of collagen fiber in the skin, bones, and ligaments. Beneficial against bone and tooth weakness. Lack of vitamin C may cause bleeding, swollen joints. Found in oranges, other citrus fruits, tomatoes, raw potatoes, raw peppers.

Vit. D - Sunshine vitamin. Essential for the assimilation of calcium, growth and development of bones, teeth, jaw formulation, maintenance of blood coagulation and cardiac rhythm. Deficiency symptoms may result in softening of bones and teeth, bone curvature in children, and calcium and phosphorous wont' absorb,

Vit. E - Essential for the assimilation of vitamins A, C, D, healthy heart and lungs, decreasing the pain in childbirth, utilization of oxygen by our tissues. Present in fresh whole grain wheat products as well as many cold-pressed vegetable oils. Deficiency symptoms may result in red blood cell breakdown, poor circulatory and muscular performance

Calcium - Essential for the transportation of nerve impulses, clotting of the blood, Vitamin C utilization, reducing cavities, formation of strong bones. Abundant in dairy products and in salmon (in the edible bones of the canned fish).

Iron - Vital component of hemoglobin, the oxygen.carrying pigment of the red blood cells. Essential for the production of energy and normal brain function. Important for stress and disease resistance. Found in liver, lean meat, eggs, and whole grain.

Magnesium - Nature uses magnesium to calm the nervous system. It is a natural sedative. May act as a catalyst in helping carbohydrates become properly assimilated instead of being stored as fat.

Manganese - Essential for normal reproductive functions, milk formulation, building resistance to disease and activating enzymes important for carbohydrate and fat production.

Niacin - Essential for the efficient use of protein. Lack of niacin results in intestinal disorders, mental depression, skin rashes. Found in liver; fish, lean meats and poultry, potatoes, nuts, and whole grains.

Potassium - Essential for balancing the system, controlling body fluids, normalizing the heartbeat, nourishing the muscles, assisting the kidneys' disposal of body waste.

Zinc - Aids in the digestion and metabolism of phosphorus and protein. Assists in burn and wound healing and in carbohydrate digestion. Essential for healthy skin.

HERBS

Alfalfa - High in chlorophyll. Excellent support for arthritis, rheumatism, colitis, ulcers, anemia, and osteoporosis.

Arnica - A first aid liniment for muscular soreness and pain from sprain, strain, over-exertion or arthritis.

Astralagus - Deep immune system tonic; improves adrenal glands function; useful in fatigue, frequent colds.

Barberry - For long-term inflammation of mouth, bleeding gums, sore throat; diarrhea from stress, excess food or dysentery.

Black Cohosh - Menstrual cramps with dull pains. Facilitates childbirth when labor delay is due to weakness, fatigue.

Burdock - Effective in dry and scaly eczema, psoriasis, acne, dandruff and boils; stimulates digestive juices.

Calendula - Internally: for peptic ulcers in remission; for varicose veins. Externally: for skin burns, healing ulcerations.

Catnip - Stimulates sweating in colds and flu. Eases stomach and intestinal cramps in children and adults.

Cayenne - Helps in viral infections, it cools dry, hot mucous membranes. Small amounts increase secretions.

Chamomile - Helps in anxiety, insomnia, indigestion, flatulence, gastritis, gingivitis, menstrual related migraines.

Chaparral - Helps in auto-immune and allergic disorders; also for people in long-term contact with chemicals, metals.

Chickweed - Externally as a rub for arthritis, strains, or gout. Useful as a diuretic for PMS water retention.

Chlorophyll - Low red blood cell count, fatigue, shortness of breath, high altitude sickness, heavy menstrual flow.

Collinsonia - Irritation of throat from intensive talking, singing, or shouting. Hemorrhoids and varicosities.

Dandelion Root - Poor bile secretion, appetite, digestive function; constipation from lack of bile; rheumatic conditions.

Devil's Claw - A safe anti-inflammatory for arthritis, rheumatism, gout, joint inflammation, and elevated cholesterol.

Dong Qual - For menopausal distress; in deficient estrogen or testosterone secretion; in PMS with dull aching pain.

Echinacea - Increases production, maturation and aggressiveness of white blood cells against intruders.

Eyebright - Internally for hay fever and allergies with watery eyes, sneezing, runny nose, stuffy sinuses.

Fennel - Eliminates flatulence. Very useful for babies with gas and distressed digestive system (e.g., diarrhea, dyspepsia).

Ginseng, Chinese Kirin Red - Most stimulating of the ginsengs. For physical or emotional stress or exhaustion.

Ginseng, Siberian - Substitute for "true" ginseng. Increases strength and endurance, resistance to infection.

Ginseng, Wild American - Emotional and physical stress, manifesting as elevated blood sugar.

Golden Seal - Helps in sub-acute or chronic mucous membranes inflammation, such as sinusitis, hay fever, allergies, gastritis.

Gotu Kola - Great support for thyroid gland where its low function contributes to emotional depression, dry skin.

Hawthorn - Helps heart irregularities with rapid heart beat episodes, or weakness of heart muscle from poor blood supply.

Hyssop - In pulmonary problems characterized by excess mucous production with difficult expectoration.

Licorice - An effective adrenal gland support. In gastric ulcers, bronchio-spasms, sore throat, painful menstruation.

Lobelia - Specific for bronchial spasms as they occur in asthma. Also, helps when trying to quit smoking.

Mullein - For coughs, especially of older asthmatic patients. Very useful in sub- acute or chronic bronchitis, emphysema.

Myrrh - in combination with Echinacea to elevate low white blood cell level. For painful ulceration of the gums or mouth.

Nettle - For hay fever. Tones up the mucous membranes especially with excessive mucous and inflammation.

Oats - Helps in the withdrawal of nicotine, cocaine or opiates. One of the best nervous system tonics available.

Pennyroyal - For late, painful, spotty menstruation accompanied by bloating, sore breasts and other PMS symptoms.

Peppermint - Stops nausea or vomiting; stimulates the production and the release of bile, prevents intestinal fermentation.

Pipsissewa - Bladder, kidney, or urethra irritation or infection especially after binging on alkaline foods, fruits.

Pleurisy Root - Useful in pleurisy, bronchitis or chest colds with dry respiratory membranes and skin.

Propolis - Mouth, gum, and intestinal infections; foul smelling diarrhea from intestinal infections.

Red Clover - High in minerals; good as a maintenance liquid during infections, hepatitis or mononucleosis.

Red Raspberry - In pregnancy, to prevent spotting in the first trimester and to increase muscle tone in the uterine walls

Red Root - Acute tonsillitis or sore throat; inflamed spleen and /or inflamed lymphatic nodes; fluid cysts in breasts, ovaries.

Sarsaparilla - Simple prostate enlargement; increases elimination of urea and uric acid. Helpful in gout, herpes.

Schizandra - Increases overall resistance. Helps fight stress, fatigue, tiredness, exhaustion and depression.

Skullcap - Inability to sleep, feeling on edge, restlessness; muscle twitching, neuralgia, sciatica.

St. John's Wort - Effective in depression, anxiety, agitation, insomnia, loss of interest and excessive sleeping.

Uva Ursi - Cystitis in paraplegics; acute cystitis and arthritis accompanied with sharp stabbing.like pain when urinating.

Valerian - Is helpful for insomnia, emotional depression, poor sleep from pain or trauma.

Yarrow - In fevers, common cold, passive bleeding of the uterus, bladder or lungs; gastric cramps, stomach gas.

Always consult with your health care practitioner. It is important to strive to find a qualified professional. Please make certain to search for the necessary expert advice and counseling for yourself.

[1] We would like to thank Life Enrichment Network for permission to reprint the section of Descriptions of Various Therapies, Herbs, Vitamins and Minerals from their Internet address earthmed.netreach.net.

SOME IMPORTANT CONTRAINDICATIONS FOR MASSAGE

You should be very careful and take a history of your clients before doing massage therapy. Many Spa's and Massage Therapists don't take the time to ask the client to fill out an Intake Form. It is imperative you know any conditions that may have a contraindication prior to giving a massage.

Here is a list of some of the contraindications for massage therapy.

LC = LOCALLY CONTRAINDICATED

Abortion (no deep abdominal work)

- Aneurysm (not even if you suspect a client who fits the profile for aneurysms)

- Appendicitis, however after appendicitis operation it can be beneficial with Dr's permission

- Acne (LC, you don't want to spread the infection)

- Advanced atherosclerosis

- Baker's cysts (LC)

- Boils (LC)

- Bronchitis (LC)

- Bunions (LC)
- Burns (LC)
- Bursitis(LC)
- Cancer (should be done only with physicians approval)
- Candidiasis (LC)
- Cirrhosis (LC in advanced stages)
- Crohn's disease: (LC, some massage with physicians supervision)
- Cysts (LC)
- Dermatitis (LC)
- Edema
- Embolism
- Encephalitis (if in acute stages
- Endometriosis (LC)
- Epilepsy (during seizures)
- Erysipelas
- Fever
- Fibroid Tumors
- Fractures (LC
- Fungal Infections (LC)
- Ganglion cysts (LC)
- Gastroenteritis (LC)
- Gout (LC)
- Headache (due to infection but indicated for tension headaches)
- Heart Attack
- Hematoma (LC)
- Hemophilia
- Hepatitis (for acute hepatitis)
- Hernia (LC)
- Herpes simplex (LC)
- Herpes zoster
- Hives (in acute stages)
- Inflammation (acute inflammation) but may be okay or subacute situations
- Interstitial cystitis (LC)

- Jaundice
- Kidney stones
- Lice and Mites
- Enlarged Liver
- Lung Cancer
- Lupus (when having acute flares and may be beneficial in subacute stages) ask Dr.
- Lyme Disease (in the acute stages)
- Lymphangitis
- Marfan's Syndrome (get physicians clearance before any massage)
- Menigitis
- Myositis Ossificans (LC)
- Neuritis (LC)
- Open Wounds/Sores (LC)
- Osteoarthritis (LC)
- Osteogenesis Imperfecti
- Ovarian cysts (LC)
- Paget's Disease
- Pelvic inflammatory disease
- Peripheral neuropathy (LC)
- Peritonitis
- Psoriasis (LC) in acute stages
- Pyelonephritis
- Renal Failure
- Rheumatoid Arthritis (during acute stages)
- Scar Tissue (LC)
- Septic Arthritis
- Sinusitis (for acute infections)
- Spasms (LC) but indicated
- Tendinitis (LC) for acute tendinitis
- Tenosynovitis (LC) in acute stages, indicated in subacute stage
- Thrombophlebitis
- Trigeminal Neuralgia (LC) in acute stage
- Torticollis (under physicians supervision)

- Tuberculosis (when active) with no infection it is okay under supervision of physician
- Ulcerative Colitis (LC) for acute stage
- Ulcers (LC)
- Urinary Tract infection (only massage when in the subacute stage)
- Varicose veins (LC) for extreme veins
- Warts (LC) remember it is possible to get warts from other people. It's a virus.
- Whiplash (in acute stages)   Indicated for subacute stage

When a name appears and has no (Local Contraindication, LC) or anything by that name it is contraindicated (Always check with a physician on any condition in question)

1.   If you have a client who sneezes often during the massage and they blow their nose into a tissue and toss it into the waste basket before leaving the treatment room and they have not washed their hands prior to opening the door, what sanitary procedure would you need to do before the next client's appointment?

You should disinfect the door knob first, and any other objects the client may have touched in the room.   Door knobs carry more germs than any other object in the room.   Always make sure you have a fresh face cover in the face cradle and it would be an excellent idea to disinfect the cradle before and after each client.

2.   True or False?   It is never a good idea to work in a dark room.
TRUE

3.   What are some of the symptoms that are associated with having a panic attack?
a) shortness of breath, b) chest pain and c) increase in heart rate

4.   TRUE OR FALSE.   If you have extended compression of the radial nerve, this can often result in radial nerve palsy. **TRUE**

5.   Yes or No. Can aluminum poisoning contribute to a possible cause for getting Alzheimer's disease?

6.   Can pancreatitis be a symptom of irritable bowel syndrome?   **NO**

7.   List at least three symptoms of rheumatoid arthritis.
Ulnar deviation deformity, morning stiffness, bilateral joint pain in your feet and hand

8.   What location does Gout most commonly occur?
      At the first metatarsophalangeal joint and around knee joints and gout is crystals deposited around joints sometime you can feel them like little marbles that roll around under the skin around the joints

9.   The xipoid process is inferior to the _____. **Pectoralis major**

10.   Define srota. **They are channels or pores according to Ayurvedic Theory.**

11.   What is the main spinal channel in Ayurvedic medicine? **Sushumna nadi**

12.   Define nadi. **They are the channels or pathways of energy where prana (ki) flows. This term is used in Ayurvedic medicine.**

13.   We have listed this question in a different way as it has been on exams and is worded differently from time to time. Question: Shiatsu is derived from _____ Japanese form of massage? **Anma**

14.   The water element consists of what yang organ in the five element theory? **The Bladder**

15.   What does Tao mean? **The law of the universe.**

16.   Acupressure points are also known as_____? **Tsubos**

17.   TRUE OR FALSE. The kidney is referred to as the foundation of yin and yang in the body? **TRUE**

18.   What is the Five Element Theory?

      Five Element Theory is one of the major systems of thought within traditional Chinese medicine. Also referred to as the "five phase" theory by some practitioners, Five Element theory has been used for more than 2,000 years as a method of diagnosis and treatment. While it is an important component of traditional Chinese medicine, today Five Element theory is not used by every acupuncturist and doctor of Oriental medicine; rather, it is employed to a certain degree, depending on the practitioner's training and education, and the style of acupuncture that he or she practices.

19.   In the five element theory, the _____element consists of muscles.
      Earth element

20.   TRUE OR FALSE. In the five element theory, the spiritual aspect of water is the will.   **TRUE**

21.   True of False. In the five element theory the water element consists of the bladder, a yang organ   **TRUE**

22.   Is the stomach associated with the earth element and referred to as a yang organ?   **YES**

23.   What is located at the base of the spine and is referred to as muladhara?   **The root charka**

24.   TRUE OR FALSE.   The governing vessel regulates all of the yin channels. **TRUE**

25.   What do charkas do?   **Control the flow of prana/energy.**

26.   What element does the heart meridian and small intestine meridian belong to?   **The fire element**

27.   What element does the triple heater meridian belong to? **The fire element**

28.   Where is the Great Eliminator (a tsubo) located? **Between the thumb and the forefinger**

29.   Define pitta.   **It is the digestion of food and metabolism of the body and is referred to as 'pitta dosha.'**

30.   What is a dosha? **It is your Ayurveda mind and body type. There are three doshas.   Vata, pitta, and kapha**

31.   Where do you apply moxibustion?   **Over the acupuncture points**

32.   Name some of the functions of the pitta dosha. **Responsible for Digestion conversions, maintains body temperature and hormonal levels, and provides heat and energy to the body, and it sharpens intellect and memory, provides color, odor, texture and luster to the skin.**

33.   What is moxibustion?   **It is a method of heating by using an herb, artemesia vulgaris.**

34.   What gland is the heart charka associated with. **The thymus gland.**

35.   Name the seven charkas.   **Crown, third eye (brow), throat, heart, solar plexus, hara, and root.**

36.   In Sports Massage, Overload is defined as what?
a) making the body work harder than normal   b) carrying too much weight than is necessary for the exercise c) Over training d) Making the body work harder than it is accustomed to working

37.   How would you define resistive movement?   **Client resists the therapist's movements at the joint.**

38.   Muscle fatigue is defined as an inability of a muscle to what? **Sustain contraction**

39.   What is known as yang or hollow organ?   **The stomach**

40.   Where is the gallbladder meridian located? **It is partially located on the lateral aspect of the hip, leg and foot.**

41.   Oriental Medicine treats the _____.   **Cause**

42.   Tsubos are also known as _____. **Trigger Points**

43.   It is the _____vessel that is a reservoir of yang energy. **Governing**

44.   It is the _____vessel that is a reservoir of yin energy. **Conception**

45.   What is the primary meridian in the back?   **The bladder meridian**

46.   Abduction of the thigh is an action of what muscles? **Gluteus medium and minimus, and the obturator internus**

47.   What nerve is the gluteus maximus innervated by? **Inferior gluteal**

48.   The _____ _____ is the most lateral muscle closest to the mastoid of the suboccipital triangle.   **Spinalis Capitis**

49.   What percentage of disease are caused by stress? 75%

50.   If a client arrives for a treatment and has a post operative scar, how long after the operation can you perform a massage? **6 months**

51.   When massaging the quadriceps which muscle is the most exterior to the outer thigh? **The vastus lateralis**

52.   If a client has very tight gastrocnemuis they may do what? **Wear high heel shoes frequently**

53.   If your client is in a prone position with a support under the abdomen, the support is used for? **Raising the back allowing the back to be massaged more easily**

54.   A client has stiff calf muscles. What would you work on? **Gastrocnemius**

55.   What is the largest organ you can massage?   **The Skin**

56.   How long do you need to be in employment before you are entitled to maternity pay?   **26 weeks**

57.   How long do you have to be in employment before you can get a 'contract for employment?'   **Two months**

58.   How often should an electrical inspection take place?   **At least once a year.**

59.   What should a 'dry' fire extinguisher not be used for?   **Fat Pan**

60.   Would advertising on TV and radio be more expensive than a newspaper ad?   **YES**

61.   How would you treat someone who has just fainted suffering from an electric shock?

62.   What would you use a UV cabinet for?   **For storage of pre sterilized equipment.**

63.   TRUE OR FALSE. Autoclave will sterilize equipment. **TRUE**

64.   What would you do if a client arrived with a medical edema? **Most edemas contraindicate circulatory massage.**

64.   What technique is known to encourage healing and better health through better posture? **ALEXANDER**

65.   What treatment uses feet as maps of body?   **Reflexology**

66.   What technique would you use if a client presents with tension in the tibialis anterior? **Effleurage**

VITAMINS AND MINERALS TO KNOW ABOUT

NUTRIENT	DEFICIENCY SYMPTOMS
Vitamin A	Night blindness, itching, dryness of the eyes
Vitamin B-1	Poor muscular and circulatory performance
Vitamin B-2	Cracks at corner of mouth, light sensitivity of eyes
Vitamin B-6	Fatigue, anemia, and hyper irritability
Vitamin B-12	Red and sore tongue, anemia and general fatigue
Vitamin C	Bruise easily, teeth and gum defects, aching joints
Vitamin D	Softening of bones and teeth
Vitamin E	Red blood cell breakdown, poor circulatory and Muscular performance
Vitamin H (biotin)	Non specific skin rash
Vitamin K	Blood won't clot

MINERALS

Calcium	Heart palpitation, weakening of bones, muscle cramps, and tooth decay

Chromium	Poor glucose intolerance
Copper	Anemia with fatigue and weakness, bone changes
Iodine	Enlarged thyroid gland in neck
Iron	Fatigue, brittle finger nails, weakness due to anemia
Magnesium	Confusion, nervousness, become angry easily
Maganese	Reproductive abnormalities
Potassium	Irregular heartbeat, muscular weakness
Selenium	Anemia, irregular heartbeat
Zinc	Slow to heal wounds, poor appetite, and loss of sense of taste

SOME COMMON BUSINESS PRACTICES TO REMEMBER

Keeping accurate records is essential to maintain a successful business. There are several reasons for keeping records. It lets you know what your expenses are; it records the progress of your business. Also your state has certain requirements you must research pertaining to taxes, licensing, etc.

Your business location is important, be zoned properly, have enough room for you and your client, a clean bathroom, clean shower, fresh linens at all times. You should have a shower in your bathroom and proper drainage in the shower. Know the difference between sole proprietorship (a business owned and operated by you alone); a partnership (combines two or more individuals); corporation (managed by several individuals/board of directors) and in a corporation the profits are shared by the stockholders. In a sole proprietorship and partnership you are responsible for the liabilities and expenses and all involvement of the business.)

There are several abbreviations you should remember.   Some help you to become more aware of body systems, as well as bodywork therapy, and muscle groups.

ABT	Asian Bodywork Therapies
AHA	American Hellerwork Association
AMA	American Medical Association
AOBTA	American Association of Bodywork Therapies of Asia
CAM	Challenge of researching Complementary and Alternative Medicine
CPT	Current Procedural Terminology. There is another abbreviation for CPT. It is Complex Physical Therapy
CRP	Constructive Rest Position
CST	Cranial Sacral Therapy
EEG	Electroencephalogram
EKG	Electrocardiogram
EMDR	Eye Movement Desensitization Repatterning
FMS	Fibromyalgia Syndrome
ICD	World Health Association's International Classification of Disease
NSAID	Non-steroidal Anti-inflammatory Drugs
SI	Structural Integration

TMC   Traditional Chinese Medicine
TAM   Traditional Asian Medicine

Piece Goods Only Go On Quilts. This statement refers to the deep lateral
    rotators and is usually named north to south as the: Periformis,
    gemellus superior, obturatur internus, gemellus inferior, obturatur
    externus and quadratus

SECTION IV

1. TRUE OR FALSE. Is it possible to drink too much water? **TRUE**

2. What is hyponatremia? **A condition caused by the dilution of sodium within the body from drinking too much water.**

3. _____ is a systematic process of gathering information. **Assessment**

4. What does a pre-event massage do for athletes? **The massage warms the body so it can help prevent injuries.**

5. Why is a post event massage recommended? **Helps to cool down the athlete's body and rid the body of possible toxins and lactic acid.**

6. List the 5 steps to the Needs Assessment when dealing with customer service with every client. **Find the need, to ensure the client feels understood, repeat back what was said; expand possibilities through up-servicing and promotional offerings; the what-why-how method of service recommendations; tell clients when you need to see them again.**

7. What makes Ayurveda unique? **It is the science based upon individuality of the client; one treatment is not right for everyone.**

8. What are trauma triggers? **They can be anything that causes energy to go through a restricted tissue area and essentially wake it up.**

9. When does REM sleep first occur? **Usually about 90 minutes after you fall asleep.**

10. TRUE OR FALSE. When there is kinesthetic dysfunction, you can not accurately sense whether certain muscles are relaxed or tense. **TRUE**

11. What are the most common types of sleep disorders? **Insomnia, narcolepsy, restless-leg-syndrome, parasomnias, obstructive sleep apnea, central sleep apnea.**

12. TRUE OR FALSE. A dysfunctional muscle will contract, but it will not return to its normal shape following contraction. **TRUE**

13.   What are the three exercises recommended in order to maintain correct posture? **The doorway stretch, the deltoid stretch, and the triceps and latissumus dorsi stretch**

14.   What stage of sleep does dreaming occur? **REM**

15.   _____ _____ is how we sense our body. **Kinesthetic awareness**

16.   What receptors in your muscles, tendons, and joints inform the brain about the position, shape, effort and direction of your body's movement? **Kinesthetic**

17.   TRUE OR FALSE.   It is relatively easy to observe and discern whether your client's breathing is functional or dysfunctional. **TRUE**

18.   How well or how poorly your breathing is, is not just a matter of how well oxygen is being supplied to your lungs, but breathing also directly influences what else? **Your mood, digestion, the efficiency of the functioning of your brain and nervous system, the balance of calcium and magnesium in your body, pain sensitivity, the tone of our muscles,   how many active trigger points you have, and how tired or alert you feel.**

19.   TRUE OR FALSE. It is important for massage therapists to understand how pharmaceutical medications might interact with massage therapy. **TRUE**

20.   The three main classes of synthetic drugs used as sedatives and hypnotics are: ____ ____ ____. **Benzodiazepine, Barbiturates, and Non benzodiazepine and non barbiturates.**

21.   List of side effects of the benzodiazepines are:
fatigue
muscle weakness
dry mouth
nausea and vomiting
dizziness
hangover effect
daytime sedation
rebound insomnia

The Adverse Effects are:
amnesia
ataxia
drug abuse
drug tolerance
drug dependence

22. List of **side effects of** barbiturates are:

drowsiness
lethargy
hypotension
vertigo
headache
nausea and vomiting
diarrhea
epigastric pain

adverse effects are:
depression
drug dependence
drug abuse
drug tolerance
hypoventilation
spasm of the larynx and bronchi
respiratory depression
allergic reaction

23. List of **side effects** of nonbenzodiazeping – nonbarbiturates

dizziness
drowsiness
lethargy
hangover effects
gastric irritation
nausea and vomiting
hypotension

Adverse effects are:

respiratory arrest
respiratory depression

24. Your massage client was involved in an auto accident and is anxious to settle the case. Your client tells you they would like to continue receiving sessions following the settlement. Should you: **Ask your client to contact their attorney so that the attorney can negotiate your fees in the settlement**

25. Your client asks you to change modalities in mid session. What would you do? **Accommodate your client's request**

26.   If a client comes in with a migraine in process what type of work would you perform? **Reike and Traditional Chinese Medicine pressure points.**

27.   Is Impetigo contagious? **YES**

28.   The pyloric valve is between which two organs? **Stomach and small intestine (duodenum)**

29.   Why is diaper draping effective? **The genitals can be discretely covered and at the same time the massage therapist is able to see and work other parts of the body.**

30.   All three hamstrings have a common origin at the ischial tuberosity. The hamstrings have a group of mucles.   Name the group of muscles that make up the hamstrings group. **Semitendinous, semimembranosus, and biceps femoris.**

31.   Muscular dystrophy is a degeneration of muscle fibers leading to: _____. **Atrophy in the skeletal muscles**

THE IMPORTANCE OF MEDICAL HISTORY FORMS

It is very important for you to have a client fill out a Medical Intake Form. When you go to a physician's office for the first time you are required to fill out a Medical History Form.

It is just as important for you to have a prospective client fill out a form before you determine if they should have a massage.

Did you know there are over 80 contraindications for massage herapy and Bodywork? There are many you should be aware of. They are listed in this book.   I have provided a sample form for you following this information. There are many reasons for having a prospective client fill out the intake form, and to interview your client to determine their needs, expectations, as well as setting your own policies and boundaries.

Some of the reasons are:

you need to explain the procedures after you have reviewed the intake form

you need to ask specific/pertinent questions

you need to listen to your clients responses

determine the type of treatment

be professional, courteous as well as sensitive

be specific about the kind of therapy/treatment

ask what you client expects from the treatment/s

be prepared to answer questions about your training, credentials and treatments

you provide and the expected results

remember to start all of your sessions with questions to determine any changes that may have occurred since their last treatment

sexual boundaries should be clearly stated

professional fees should be stated prior to any treatments

clearly state what your policy is for i.e. canceled and/or late appointments

[SAMPLE] MASSAGE THERAPY AND BODYWORK INTAKE FORM

Name_____

Date_____

Address_____Telephone_____

City/State/Zip_____Business_____

Occupation_____ SS#_____

Male_____ Female_____

Is Mother living? _____ Is Father living?_____

How did you find out about my service?_____

Was there a specific reason for seeking massage therapy?_____

Have you have massage treatments before?_____

If so, by whom?_____

What is your reason for desiring massage treatments?_____

Were you referred by someone?_____

By whom?_____

How would you describe you describe your general health?_____

Are you currently under a health care professional/s? _____ If so, please

list them. Name_____Name_____

Phone Numbers:_____ _____

Are you currently taking any medication? _____If so, list all medications including

hormone replacement therapy, Aspirin, Advil, herbs, and any over the counter pills,

etc._____

_____

May I have permission to contact your health care professional/s, therapist/s for

further evaluation? _____

Have you had any serious operations, traumatic accidents, chronic illness, chronic

pain, chronic virus infections, and have you been under the care of a psychotherapist,

psychiatrist, counselor, in the past twelve months?_____ If so, please be

specific._____

_____

Has there been any history of the following in your family?

Heart problems_____ If so, who?_____

Diabetes_____ If so, who?_____

High blood pressure _____ If so, who?_____

Low blood pressure_____ If so, who?_____

Arthritis _____ If so, who?_____

Depression _____ If so, who?_____

Cancer _____ If so, who?_____

Have you ever been tested for HIV and if so when?_____

In case of an emergency who would I notify?

Name_____ Phone No/s: (   ) _____

Address_____ Phone No/s: (   ) _____

City/State/Zip_____

Have you had any of the following within the past three to four months? There are

contraindications for these maladies.   Please place a check by each one that would

apply.

LC beside a condition would indicate (Locally contraindicated)

Abortion (no deep abdominal work)

Aneurysm (not even if you suspect a client who fits the profile for aneurysms)

Appendicitis, however after appendicitis operation it can be beneficial with Dr's

Permission

Acne (LC, you don't want to spread the infection)
- Advanced atherosclerosis
- Baker's cysts (LC)
- Boils (LC)
- Bronchitis (LC)
- Bunions (LC)
- Burns (LC)
- Bursitis(LC)
- Cancer (should be done only with physicians approval)
- Cirrhosis (LC in advanced stages)
- Crohn's disease: (LC, some massage with physicians supervision)
- Cysts (LC)
- Dermatitis (LC)
- Ovarian cysts (LC)
- Paget's Disease
- Pelvic inflammatory disease
- Peripheral neuropathy (LC)
- Peritonitis
- Psoriasis (LC) in acute stages
- Pyelonephritis
- Renal Failure
- Rheumatoid Arthritis (during acute stages)
- Scar Tissue (LC)
- Septic Arthritis
- Sinusitis (for acute infections)
- Spasms (LC) but indicated
- Tendinitis (LC) for acute tendinitis
- Tenosynovitis (LC) in acute stages, indicated in subacute stage
- Thrombophlebitis
- Trigeminal Neuralgia (LC) in acute stage
- Torticollis (under physician's supervision)
- Tuberculosis (when active) with no infection it is okay under supervision of physician
- Ulcerative Colitis (LC) for acute stage
- Ulcers (LC)
- Urinary Tract infection (only massage when in the subacute stage)
- Varicose veins (LC) for extreme veins
- Warts (LC) remember it is possible to get warts from other people. It's a virus.
- Whiplash (in acute stages)   Indicated for subacute stage

When a name appears and has no (Local Contraindication, LC) or anything by that name it is contraindicated (Always check with a physician on any condition in question)

I have filled out the Intake Form to be best of my ability and understand that massage therapy treatments are not meant to replace a Doctor's treatment. I also understand that massage and bodywork treatments are considered to be an additional aid in the helping me to improve and/or maintain a healthy body. I have been told by the therapist that all information discussed during treatments is to remain confidential. I also understand if I fail to cancel any appointments 24 hours prior to a scheduled appointment, I will be responsible for paying the full fee. If an emergency prevents my calling to cancel I understand I will not be charged.

Signature_____ Date_____
THIS IS JUST A SAMPLE FORM AND YOU MAY WANT TO IMPROVISE

SECTION V

1. In reflexology treatments, what area on the foot would have the pressure point relating to the neck in treatment? **big toe, base of big toe**
2. In massage treatment is it a general practice to massage by muscle groups? **YES**
3. Is the back effleuraged before petrissage movement? **YES**
4. Should you always be in a standing position while massaging a patient? **NO**
5. What is Aroma Therapy? **Various scents which are added to massage lubricants or used in a vapor type of machine, which has either a stimulating or relaxing effect**
6. What are meridians and how many regular meridians are there? **Oriental philosophy/medical science believe that meridians are a system of pathways or channels pertaining to energy (ki) that circulates in a network of channels and collateral in the body. There are 12 regular or main meridians.**
7. Name at least 4 benefits of good posture. **Improves circulation, appearance, prevents fatigue and backaches, and better on your muscles and joints**
8. Where did Yoga originate? **India**
9. It is important to exercise when dieting for weight loss, and if so give the reason why? **Yes, because it firms as well as proportions the body as it burns calories**
10. What is one of the most popular forms of exercise and list at least 2 benefits? **Walking, because there is no equipment required. It improves your circulation.**
11. What is TMJ dysfunction and how can you treat it? **TMJ is temporomandibular joint. The mandibular, which plays an important role in jaw pain, has muscles that are attached to the mandibular and if there are spasms in this area the jaw point (in pressure point therapy) can well respond to pressure**.
12. What is torticollis? Latin term for twisted neck. **(tortus) twisted and (collis) neck**
13. What are some of the benefits of lymphatic massage/drainage? **Purifies and regenerates tissues, expedites the balance of the body's internal chemistry, helps to balance the functions of all body organs as well as the immune system.**
14. TRUE OR FALSE. Damaged tissue can be carried away during massage, and circulation of blood enables the nutrients to enter the damaged area helping the healing process. **TRUE**
15. What role do the liver, pancreas, and glands in the small intestine play in the digestion process? **They supply digestive secretions.**

16. Define pathogenic. **It is harmful bacteria.**
17. What is the longest muscle in the body, and where is it located? **sartorius -located in the leg (thigh)**
18. Give the definition of a bone. **A bone is a form of dense connective tissue which supports the muscles of the body and protects delicate internal structures, and produces blood cells.**
19. What is Reflexology? **Reflexology is the application of applying pressure to a reflex point (usually on the hands and feet) to relieve tension and, improve blood supply to certain regions of the body to help normalize body functions.**
20. What do enzymes do? **Aid in digestion**
21. Name some of the benefits of a facial massage. **Helps to keep the muscles toned, increases circulation of blood, and keeps the oil and sweat glands functioning properly.**
22. Describe what a centripetal movement is. **A centripetal movement is a strong pressure directed towards a center i.e. the heart and it follows the direction of the blood current.**
23. TRUE OR FALSE. Light rays are very beneficial in the treatment of varicose veins. **FALSE**
24. Define ligament. **Connective tissue connecting bones to bones**
25. TRUE OR FALSE. Diastolic is a higher reading than systolic. **False**
26. Name at least 4 ethical codes pertaining to massage therapy. **have a good understanding of massage, keep your appointments, do not take advantage of client, explain the draping to the client before the massage.**
27. Name the 3 arches in the foot. **transverse, medial longitudinal, and lateral**
28. What is a catheter? **A tube for fluids**
29. What are the 4 basic movements used in massage therapy and name the various forms/names of these movements?
    (1)   percussion =slapping , tapping, cupping, hacking beating
    (2)   compression = petrissage /friction/vibration
    (3)   joint = passive and active movements
    (4)   effleurage = stroking with palm of hand or fingertips
    Note: Tapotement is also referred to as a tapping movement
30. Describe what a "passive movement" means in massage. **it is when the joints are massaged and the client does not have to actively move their muscles**
31. In massage therapy, what is the meaning of "contraindication"? **It would not be advisable to massage because of the client's condition and massage might be harmful more than helpful**
32. Name 3 forms of harmful bacteria. **spirilla, bacilli and cocci**
33. What is Shiatsu? **Shiatsu is a treatment whereby you apply pressure with the ball of your thumb along the meridians to increase circulation.**
34. What is Zygote? What is the zygomatic process? **Zygote is fertilized ovum. Zygomatic process is the process of the temporal or squamosal bone helping to form the zygomatic arch.**
35. What are the gonads? **sex glands (the ovaries and testes)**
36. Name the 3 separate bones of the hip bone. **ilium, ischium, and pubis**

37. TRUE OR FALSE. The brain is the vital force that controls all the body functions. **TRUE**

38. Name the four general classifications of bones and give one example of each. **long = femur, short = patella, irregular = vertebrae, and flat= scapula**

39. TRUE OR FALSE. The nerves are the vital force that activates all muscle functions. **TRUE**

40. Give the basic principles for draping a client. **Any tight clothing should be removed first of all, and either a towel or sheet should be used to cover the parts of the body that are not being massaged. It is important to make sure that the client is not embarrassed or exposed unnecessarily. The purpose is for the client to be comfortable, relaxed and at ease. All of your movements should be very businesslike.**

41. Please be specific in describing how you would drape a female client using the "top cover method". **When the client is on the table have the top cover (can be either a large sheet, or large bath towel), cover the client lengthwise covering the entire body all but the head. When you massage the arm you would fold the top cover exposing only the area that you are massaging. When you massage the leg, you would tuck the cover under the opposite leg positioning the cover tightly (but not too tight) along the inguinal crease.**

42. Describe the diaper draping method in detail. **You would use a very large towel (terry towel preferably) for covering the chest and long enough to come to a little bit above the knees of the client. You would then fold the end of the towel (end just above the knees) intofour smooth folds. These folds taper to fit the contours of the body. The clients leg would then be raised enough to allow the end of the towel to be tucked under the sacrum. The client is then draped properly.**

43. Describe in detail how you would drape a female client properly before you would begin an abdominal massage. **You would fold another towel (in additional to the one covering the body) to cover the breasts and place it over the first towel. Then you would pull the first towel down while you hold the folded towel and place it over the breasts. Then you would take the original first cover of the client and fold the top of this first towel across the client's pelvic area. Then you would raise the client's arm and then tuck the towel (the folded one for the breasts) and tuck this securely under the scapula. Then you would put the client's arm down and follow the same procedure for the other arm, etc.**

44. How are cold applications beneficial? **stimulates the nerves - increases movement of body cells - improves your circulation**

45. Name one benefit of a hot water treatment. **Increases circulation of blood to the surface of the skin**

46.   Name the organs of the respiratory system. **lungs, bronchial tubes, trachea, nose, and mouth**

47.   What is another name for the trachea? **windpipe**

48.   What is Fascia? **A tough connective tissue that has an elastic component and a matrix that is a gelatinous like substance.**

49.   What is Myofascial Release? **A hands-on technique that applies prolonged light pressure with specific directions into the fascia system.**

50.   How many bones are found in the upper leg and give the names of these bones? **One. The Femur**

51.   Is it really necessary to get a medical record of a client? **YES**

52.   In Sports/Athletic massage, what are the major applications? **Massage before, during and after an event and also during any rehabilitation**

53.   What are the connecting links between arteries and veins called? **capillaries**

54.   Name the five divisions of the spine. **cervical vertebrae, thoracic vertebrae, lumbar vertebrae, sacrum vertebrae, and the coccygeal vertebrae (also called the coccyx)**

55.   Define what muscle tone is. **When muscle fibers are constantly in a state of slight contraction.**

56.   What part of the body is the Achilles Tendon located? **Just above the heel**

57.   List at least 3 things a massage therapist should do in order to maintain hygiene and sanitation. **wash hands before and after each treatment, keep nails short and trimmed so that you won't scratch a client, have clean sheets, linens, and towels available for each client, and change linens after each treatment**

58.   Define tissue. **A group or collection of cells which act together in the performance of a particular function.**

59.   Define Anatomy. **Anatomy is the study of the structure of the body.**

60.   Define Physiology? **Physiology is the study of the functions of the body.**

61.   Where does the digestion of proteins begin turning into amino acids? **in the stomach**

62.   Describe what "active movement" is in massage therapy. **The client participates in the exercises in which the voluntary muscles are contracted.**

63.   What is Acupuncture and what is an integral part of this type of treatment? **Acupuncture is a treatment where the skin is punctured with needles along certain meridians of the body for therapeutic purposes.**

64.   Name at least 14 other body therapies or specialized massage techniques other than Swedish massage therapy. **Rolfing, Feldenkrais, Myofascial Release, Reiki, Trager, Shiatsu, Deep Tissue Technique (Athletic/Sports), Reflexology, Lymphatic Drainage, Structural Integration, Polarity, Acupressure, Cranial Sacral Therapy, Jin Shin Do.**

65.   What is hydrotherapy? **Water treatments for the external part of the body.**

66.   When are salt rubs given? Anytime or following a cabinet bath or hot bath

67.   How high can a temperature be in a steam vapor? **140 degrees Fahrenheit**

68.   TRUE OR FALSE. The skin can safely tolerate 120 degrees Fahrenheit. **FALSE.** 110 degrees Fahrenheit

69.   Name at least 10 parts of the body involved in the process of digestion. **Teeth, tongue, salivary glands, mouth, stomach, liver, gallbladder, pancreas, small intestine and gastric glands**

70.   Name a couple of contraindications in Sports/Athletic massage. **Injury, illness or any abnormal condition**

71.   Name the various massage movements that have a stimulating effect on the nervous system. **Vibration, friction, and percussive movements**

72.   What can Structural Integration do? **It can endeavor to bring the physical composition of the body into alignment and balance around a central axis.**

73.   Can massage relieve anxiety? **YES**

74.   What muscles can cross both the hip and the knee and act on both joints? **The hamstrings**

75.   Name 4 gastrointestinal disorders. **constipation - ulcers - spastic colon - irritable bowel syndrome**

76.   What is impetigo? **A skin infection that could be caused by strep or staph.**

77.   What is reflexology? **It is the application of applying pressure to a reflex point (usually on the hands, feet) to relieve tension, improve the blood supply to certain regions of the body to help normalize body functions.**

78.   What is Rolfing and what is one benefit of having Rolfing treatments? **Rolfing is a method of structural integration, and a deep connective tissue massage. One benefit is that it increases suppleness of the muscles.**

79.   TRUE OR FALSE. Nonpathogenic bacteria are also harmful. **False. sometimes they are helpful**

80.   What function does the diaphragm perform? **aids in the expansion of the thoracic cavity and contraction of the lungs**

81.   Why should the massage therapist explain the draping technique to their client? **It prevents embarrassment to the client as well as the therapist.**

82.   In what part of the body are starches digested into the sugar stage? **the mouth**

83.   What are some of the things that can be relieved by applying shiatsu? **Insomnia, high blood pressure, headaches, nervous tension, sore muscles, constipation.**

84.   What does Shiatsu mean? **pressure of the finger - broken down it means (finger/shi) (atsu/pressure)**

85.   In sports/athletic massage what are the goals of the pre-event massage and the goals for the post-event massage? **Goal for the pre-event massage is to increase the flexibility and circulation in the areas of the body that are going to be used; the goal in the post-event massage is to increase the circulation in order to clear out the metabolic wastes, to quite the nervous system and to reduce any muscle spasms and/or tension.**

86.   Describe what a Centrifugal movement is. **A movement away from the center causing a decrease in the flow of blood lessening pressure to the heart.**

87.   In heat and lamp treatments what are the 3 rays used? **Ultraviolet, visible light and infrared**

88.   Name one thing that is very important for the massage therapist to do in order to avoid fatigue and backache during treatment? **Pay attention to good posture and make sure that the massage table is at the proper level for the therapists height.**

89.   TRUE OR FALSE. One of the benefits of a whirlpool bath is a decrease in blood circulation. **FALSE - there is an increase**

90.   What is a pore, sometimes referred to as a follicle? **A minute opening of the sweat glands on the surface of the skin.**

91.   What are the 2 types of bone tissue? **Compact and spongy**

92.   TRUE OR FALSE. Bones receive nourishment through blood vessels that enter through the periosteum into the interior of the bone. **TRUE**

93.   TRUE OR FALSE. A lesion is a structural change in the tissue and can be caused by either injury or disease. **TRUE**

94.   Can massage relieve anxiety?   **YES**

95.   What percentage of an adult's body weight is skeletal muscle? **40%**

96.   What 3 main techniques are used in acupressure? **Pressing the pressure points, touching and rubbing these pressure points**

97.   Where did acupuncture originate? **China**

98.   What is the main cause of foot problems today? **Wearing shoes that are not fitted properly.**

99.   Sports massage is also referred to what other name? **Athletic Massage**

100.   Name a massage movement/technique that has a calming effect on the nervous system.   **Petrissage - light effleurage or a very gentle stroking and light friction**

101.   What should the temperature be in your massage therapy room? **75 to 80 degrees F.**

102.   What is lymphangiitis? **Blood poisoning or inflammation of the lymphatic vessels**

103.   Define Pathology. **The part of medicine that is concerned with the structural and functional changes caused by disease.**

104.   Name the 3 sections of the spine. **cervical - thoracic - lumbar**

105.   Name 3 skeletal dysfunctions. **lordosis (swayback) - scoliosis (an abnormality of the spine with pain) - kyphosis (humpback)**

106.   What lubricates the joints? **synovial fluid**

107.   What purpose does cartilage and ligaments serve? **List the purpose of cartilage first. Cartilage cushions the bones at joints i.e. preventing jarring between bones, and gives shape to the external features on the body i.e. your ear and nose. Ligaments help support bones at the joints i.e. the wrist.**

108.   What is fossa? **a depression**

109.   What is sebum? **The oily secretion/substance that comes from the sebaceous gland.**

110.   What is sinus? **a cavity within a bone**

111.   Name one function of bone marrow. **Bone marrow helps in the nutrition of the bone**

112. TRUE OR FALSE. A very effective way to bring blood to an area is through the application of ice. **True**
113. Define a duct. **a canal for fluids**
114. What are the appendages of the skin? **nails -hair and also the sweat/oil glands**
115. Name a joint that is immovable. **Synarthrotic**
116. How would you massage over the bones? **You would follow the form of the bones very carefully.**
117. What muscle opens the eye? **the levator palpabrae superioris muscle**
118. What are the 10 most important systems of the body? **nervous - skeletal - respiratory - reproductive - digestive - circulatory - muscular - endocrine - integumentary and excretory system**
119. The urinary system is part of what system? **excretory system**
120. The blood vascular and lymph vascular is part of what system? **circulatory system**
121. What is a clear, yellow fluid that bathes cells? **Interstitial fluid associated with lymph**
122. What are the 4 main anatomic parts of the body? **the extremities, trunk, spine and head**
123. What does integument mean? **skin or covering**
124. A patient comes to you and had just sprained their ankle. There is considerable swelling and a lot of pain. What type of treatment would you give? **Massage above and below the area in an attempt to reduce the swelling and help alleviate the pain.**
125. A elderly woman has had arthritis of the spine for several years and she stands in a slightly flexed position. When she tries to stand in a normal position there is a lot of pain. What type of treatment would you give? **Massage to relieve pain and any spasms and also moist heat packs.**
126. A violinist is recovering from surgery for Carpal Tunnel Syndrome. Her left hand is very painful. The finger flexors are stiff and she is having a very hard time using her hand. What type of treatment would you give? **Exercise to assist her in regaining use of her hand, massage, and heat treatments**
127. What is meant by reflex effects? **When your hands stimulate the sensory receptors of the skin and subcutaneous tissues it causes reflex effects. Example: Lymphatic flow is an effect of deep pressure treatments by stroking or compression movements.**
128. What is meant by venostasis (syn: phlebostasis) and list three contraindications when you would not massage situations showing venostasis? **It is a condition that develops due to muscular inactivity whereby gravity inhibits the normal venous return towards the heart. You would not massage if there is a possibility of spreading inflammation, possibility of dislodging a thrombus, or if there is this type of obstruction that the assistance of massage would not improve the venous flow.**
129. How do muscles maintain a metabolic balance? **Usually through normal activity...when they contract they get rid of toxic products.**

130. Define edema and 3-4 causes of edema. **Edema is excess interstitial fluid in the tissues, aka swelling. (1) increased resistance to outflow at the venous end of the capillary bed, (2) decreased resistance to flow through the arterioles and capillary sphincters that supply the capillary bed, and (3) increased gravitational forces.**

131. Will massage reduce obesity? **NO**

132. Can massage take the place of active exercise. **NO**

133. What is a hematoma? **A swelling that contains blood.**

134. How many ribs are there in the body? **24**

135. Define condyle. **A rounded knuckle, or articular surface like prominence usually at a point of articulation or at the extremity of a bone.**

136. What are bursae? **Little sacks lined with synovial membrane and lubricated with synovial fluid.**

137 List the movements of the diarthric joints. **Gliding, pivoting, saddle, ball and socket, hinge movements**

138 Internal rotation means to move where? **Medially or toward the midline**

139. External rotation means to move where? **Laterally or away from midline**

140. Hyperextension movement means what? **to increase the angle beyond the anatomical position**

141 What does flexion mean? **to decrease the angle at a joint**

142. What does extension mean? **to increase the angle at a joint**

143. What does circumduction mean? **to move the distal end of an extremity in a circle while the proximal end remains fixed**

144 What does adduction mean? **to move a part toward the midline**

145. What does dorsiflexion mean? **to move the foot upward**

146. What does plantar flexion mean? **to move the foot downward (to extend downward)**

147. What does inversion mean? **to turn the plantar surface toward the midline**

148. What does eversion mean? **to turn the plantar surface away from the midline**

149. What does pronation mean? **to move the palm downward**

150. What does protraction mean? **to move a part of the body forward**

151. What does depression (in movement) mean? **to lower a part of the body**

152. What is fibromylasia? **a disorder - the musculoskeletal function throwing the neurovascular system "off balance". Many factors that can precipitate it are personality, disordered sleep patterns, occupation, hobbies, posture, weather, etc.**

153. **What is the difference between asthma and bronchitis? Asthma is a panting - paroxysmal dyspnea accompanied by the adventitious sounds caused by a spasm of the bronchial tubes or due to swelling of their mucous membrane. Bronchitis is the inflammation of bronchial mucous membranes.**

154. List the difference between neuralgia and neuritis. **Neuralgia is acute pain extending along the course of one or more nerves, and neuritis is inflammation of a nerve/s usually associated with a degenerative process.**

155. What causes a duodenal ulcer? **action of gastric juices**
156. Define what colitis/spastic colon is.
It is inflammation of the colon, attacks occur spasmodically accompanied by constipation. Spastic, colicky pain in mid-abdomen. Tenacious, gelatinous mucus and shreds of mucous membrane may be passed.
157. List some of the things that you want to ask in your interviewing a new patient.
Did a physician suggest treatments, have you had any injuries, accidents, etc. and be sure and cover all things that may be a contraindication to treatment before you start a massage. Take temperature before treatment, and ask for a complete medical history so you will know if there is high blood pressure, ulcers, etc.
158. Define what is the origin of a muscle and what is the insertion of a muscle.
The more proximal attachment site of a muscle is referred to as the origin, and the more distal attachment site of a muscle is called the insertion.
159. Name two endangerment sites on the body.
Popliteal fossa and femoral triangle
160. Tell why it is important that once you start a treatment that it not be interrupted.
You do not want to interrupt any flow of rhythm or cause the patient to become disturbed in anyway.
161. Name 6 functions of the skin.
protects the body - regulates the temperature - acts as a excretory and secretory organ - oxygen is taken in and carbon dioxide is discharged through the process called respiration - and -absorption
162. How many bones are in the adult human body and be specific i.e. **EXAMPLE: lower extremities (62 bones)?**
spine = vertebrae 26 bones, head = face (14) cranium (8) ear (6) hyoid bone (1) 26 bones, thorax = ribs and sternum 25 bones, and the upper extremities 64 bones.
163. List 3 things that compose the skeletal system.
ligaments -bones - cartilage
164. What is the largest organ of the body?
the skin
165. Name two main layers of the skin.
dermis & epidermis
166. What are the layers of the epidermis and the epidermis of the palms and soles?
the mucosum, granulosum, lucidum, and stratum corneum, and the palms and soles have the following strata: stratum corneum, stratum lucidum, stratum granulosum, stratum spinosum), and stratum gasale, and the other parts of the body, the stratum lucidum may be absent in some cases.
167. What are the 2 major glands in the skin and tell what the function is of these glands?
sebaceous = secrete sebum, and sudoriferous = excretes sweat

168. List one of the goals in receiving Rolfing treatments.
to reshape the body's physical posture as well as to realign the muscular and connective tissue.

169. List the inorganic matter found in bones.
calcium carbonate and calcium phosphate

170. List the organic matter found in bones.
marrow - blood vessels - bone cells

171. What is periosteum?
It is the protective covering of the bone

172. Define joints.
Joints are the connections between the surfaces of bones.

173. How do most massage therapists begin a massage?
Generally with the client in a face up position unless the client prefers the prone position

174. Name some contraindications in massage.
abnormal body temperature, infectious disease, varicose veins, phlebitis, aneurosa, high blood pressure, edema, cancer (in extreme conditions recovering from radiation treatment, however; massage is wonderful for cancer patients but should be done by someone who is trained in this area), intoxication, chronic fatigue, psychosis, hernia

175. Name the 12 cranial nerves.
**olfactory
hypoglossal
spinal accessory
optic
oculomotor
facial
acoustic/auditory
vagus/pneumogastric
trochlear
trigeminal/trifacial
glossopharyngeal
abducent**

176. What is the first thing that you would do if you suspected a heart attack? **Place the individual in a comfortable position**

177. Would you use cold applications in the treatment of tendonitis?   **YES**

178. What is the largest organ and gland in the body? **Liver**

179. List the effects of percussion.
**breaks up adhesions and reduces scar tissue
aids in shedding of dead skin cells and reduces blemishes
increases range of motion and strengthens muscle
tones the muscles and stimulates circulation
tones muscles/stimulates circulation**

180. *TRUE OR FALSE.* Friction massage movement is used to break down the adhesions of a well-healed scar. **TRUE**

181. Which joint can only move back and forth? The Knee Joint

182. Name a flexors of the hip. **Iliopsoas (inner hip muscles)**
183. Define what a Trager session consists of.
    Is it a gentle rocking and the movement of muscles, limbs, and joints in order to produce sensory experiences of freedom, ease, and lightness. The therapist uses their hands and mind to communicate a positive experience through the patient's tissue to the central nervous system.
184. Define Yin/Yang.
    Yin/Yang is a Buddhist theory that demonstrates the natural process of continuous change where nothing is of itself, but is seen as aspects of the whole or as two opposites, yet is complementary aspects of existence itself.
185. How long should you take a hot bath?
    No longer than 20 minutes maximum
186. The heart, blood vessels including the arteries, veins, and capillaries are the main part of what?
    The blood-vascular system
187. What is the usual order of massage movements and list these in order?
    Begins with arms (if the client prefers) or back otherwise, then front of legs, chest, neck, and abdomen.
188. What is the name of the main artery of the body? **Aorta**
189. Should a client be advised to drink plenty of water after a massage treatment and if so explain why or why not?
    Yes, the system needs to be washed out because you have stimulated the flow of blood, and your body needs the water to flush out the toxins.
190. Name the functions of the following in their order: veins, heart, arteries, and capillaries.
    Veins carry impure blood from the capillaries back to the heart; heart function keeps the blood moving through the body; arteries carry purified blood from the heart to the capillaries; and the capillaries bring nourishment to the cells as well as remove waste products.
191. Plasma, red corpuscles, platelets, and white corpuscles are found where?
    In the blood
192. What artery supplies blood to the chest, arm, and shoulder? **axillary artery**
193. What muscle moves the scalp? **Epicranius**
194. What does the masseter muscle do? **Raises the lower jaw**
195. What is the principal large artery on the right side of the neck? **right carotid artery**
196. What is the function of the pulmonary artery?
    Divides into left and right branches and takes the blood into the lungs
197. Venous blood is carried through which artery up to the lungs to be oxygenated and purified? **Pulmonary artery**

198.	There are two sets of nerves that regulate the heartbeat. What are they?
	Sympathetic and the vagus nerves

199.	Define lacteals.
	They carry chyme from the intestine to the thoracic duct.

200.	What is phlebitis?
	Inflammation of a vein accompanied by swelling and pain

201.	What is osteoporosis?
	A disease in which there is a decrease in bone density

202.	What three groups of muscles make up the hamstrings?
	The posterior thigh (the long head of biceps femoris, semi-membranosus, and semi tendinosus)

203.	What are the gluteals? **The muscles of the buttocks**

204.	Name at lease 6 lubricants that are used in therapy.
	cocoa butter (used on scar tissue), 70% alcohol (good for stump ends), powder, mineral oil/baby oil, lanolin based cold cream, vegetable oil/olive oil (good for baby massage or for anyone that can use the extra nutrients)

205.	What type of treatment would you give to someone who has just had a cast removed after having surgery to relieve recurrent shoulder dislocation?
	tapotement, effleurage, and petrissage to deltoid and trapezius in an attempt to increase the circulation and relieve spasm

206.	What type of treatment would you give to a patient who has had severe bursitis in the left shoulder for 2 years?
	Heat, massage, and exercise to the left shoulder

207.	For a patient who has severe lower back pain from a herniated disc with severe sciatica, and whenever there are any movements from the right leg which stretches the sciatic nerve, it is very painful. What type of treatment would you give?
	petrissage to the lower back area to help relieve the pain however, it might be a good idea to suggest they see a D.O. if they don't already have one.

208.	Tell what the following muscles do:
	(a) serratus anterior
	(b) obliquus capitis inferior
	(c) rectus abdominis
	(d) trapezius
	(e) sacrospinalis
	(f) obliquus capitis superior
	(g) longus colli
	(h) quadratus lumborum
	(i) latissimus dorsi
	(j) sartorius
	(k) pectoralis major
	(l) pectoralis minor
	(m) intercostales externi
	(n) levatores costarum
	(o) diaphragm
	(p) temporalis
	(q) recti muscles
	(s) psoas major

(t) rhomboid
(u) infra-spinatus
(v) supra-spinatus
(w) deltoid
(x) teres minor
(y) teres major
(z) triceps brachialis

Answers

(a) raises ribs in breathing
(b) rotates cranium
(c) compresses the abdomen
(d) draws head backward
(e) keeps your spine erect
(f) draws head backward
(g) rotates the spine
(h) bends the trunk of body
(i) draws arm backward
(j) rotates thigh outward and leg inward, bends leg/thigh
(k) draws arm forward and downward
(l) depresses point of shoulder
(m) stretches the chest during breathing
(n) raises the ribs during breathing
(o) main muscle of respiration
(p) raises the lower jaw and presses it against the upper jaw
(q) rotates your eyeball
(r) bends your head to one side and forward
(s) bends trunk on thigh or thigh on trunk
(t) draws shoulder blade backward and upward
(u) rotates arm outwardly
(v) helps to raise the arm side ward
(w) extends and bends the arm
(x) rotates humerus outward
(y) assists in drawing humerus downward and backward
(z) extends the forearm

209. What are muscles attached to?
tendons
210. What is a characteristic of a amphiarthrotic joint?
It has limited motion, movable and non moveable.
211. Define fascia.
connective tissue covering muscles and separating their layers or groups of layers
212. What is the difference between diarthrotic and synarthrotic joints?
Synarthrotic joints are very limited and diarthrotic joints are freely movable.
213. There are two divisions of the autonomic nervous systems, the sympathetic and the parasympathetic. Which of these expands energy? **the sympathetic**
214. How many pairs of cranial nerves are there and how many pairs of spinal nerves are there?
12 pairs cranial and 31 pairs spinal
215. The ulnar nerve supplies what two joints?
elbow and shoulder joints

216.   The pneumogastric nerve supplies what?
       the heart and lungs
217.   The greater occipital nerve supplies what?
       the back of the neck
218.   The intercostal nerve supplies what?
       the upper abdomen
219.   What does the sacral nerve supply?
       the muscles and skin of the lower extremities
220.   What nerve supplies the hip and knee joints?
       the obturator nerve
221.   What are hormones?
       the secretions manufactured by the endocrine glands
222.   Where is the pituitary gland located?
       just behind the point of the optic nerve crossing in the brain
223.   Name the important endocrine glands.
       pituitary, adrenal, sex glands, thyroid, pancreas
224.   What are the two divisions of the vascular system?
       **blood vascular system (heart and blood vessels) and the lymph
       vascular system (lymph glands and lymphatics)**
225.   Name two diseases of the blood?
       hemophilia and anemia
226.   The right atrium of the heart receives impure blood from the what?
       vena cava
227.   Veins of the abdomen, lower extremities and pelvis empty into what
       vein? **inferior vena cava**
228.   Which ventricle does the aorta send blood to all parts of the body
       except the lungs? **the left ventricle**
229.   What is the name of the large artery on the left side of the neck? **the
       left carotid artery**
230.   The left atrium receives purified blood through what vein?
       pulmonary vein
231.   The veins from the neck, head, thorax and upper extremities empty
       into what vein? **superior vena cava**
232.   What does the pulmonary artery do? **it conveys venous blood from
       the right ventricle to the lungs**
233.   What is meant by sanitation? **cleanliness**
234.   How many bones form the wrist and what are their names?
       eight bones called carpal
235.   In massage of the lower extremities, the manipulations are applied in
       what sequence? **effleurage, tapotement, friction, and nerve
       strokes**
236.   Why is massage of the chest muscles beneficial?
       **Because you are helping the muscles that assist in respiration,
       and in this way you will be indirectly helping the lungs to
       perform their function. It also activates muscles that assist the
       movements of the arm, as well as that of the shoulders.**
237.   Why should the client's knees be flexed for abdominal massage?
       to relax the abdominal muscles
238.   What areas of the body have the thickest skin?
       the palms of hands and soles of feet

239. What is a "Charley Horse" and how can it be avoided in applying massage?
It is a spastic muscle contraction and can be avoided by not hacking across the muscle.

240. How much pressure should be applied in friction of the thigh muscles?
enough pressure to move the underlying muscles

241. How does massage applied to the spinal area improve the bodily functions?
It activates the nerves and brings fresh blood to stimulate and nourish the nerves, which branching out from this area are the means used by the brain to carry messages throughout the body.

242. When pressure is applied on the seventh cranial nerve what muscles are activated? **the facial muscles**

243. What is meant by the therapeutic field in hydrotherapy?
treatment of condition by use of water

244. What is used in a saline bath? common salt

245. Describe a twisting manipulation that is applied to the muscles?
You place both of your hands next to each other and push the tissue forward with the palm of one hand as the fingers of the other hand pull the tissue back.

246. Define the term "remedial exercises".
It is the application of body movements that maintain or restore normal muscle and joint function.

247. How can the therapist avoid straining a joint?
by knowing the types of movements that each joint is capable of performing

248 Why should the therapist avoid the "hacking" transversely across the muscles?   **It could cause a Charley Horse.**

249. Percussion massage is used more on what parts of the body?
buttocks, thighs, and areas that are heavily muscled

250. Would you use the hacking motion over the tibia?   **No**

251. Name the two movements that the shoulder cannot perform.
supination and pronation

252. Explain why you would not want to over stimulate a weak muscle during massage. **It could cause muscle strain and could create some toxic poison.**

253. What is epistaxis? **a nose bleed**

254. How do you know if you have used too much oil in a massage treatment? **because your movements will be difficult**

255. What is tonic contraction?
Sustained partial contraction of some of a skeletal muscle in response to stretch receptors is called a tone, or tonic contraction.

256. What is isotonic? What is isometric contraction?
Isotonic is having the same tension, tone or pressure.
Isometric contraction is the contraction of a muscle in which shortening of the muscle is prevented, and tension is developed and does not result in body movement.

257. TRUE OR FALSE. Claustrophobia is a fear of heights.
False.   It is a fear of being confined in a small space.

258.   TRUE OR FALSE. Agoraphobia is a dread or fear of crowds of people. **TRUE**

259.   Give another name for the Lingual Bone. **hyoid bone**

260.   What is the difference between peritoneum and periosteum? **Periosteum is the membrane that covers the bones and peritoneum is a closed sac composed of a thin sheet of elastic and fibrous tissue that lines the abdominal cavity.**

261.   Give the normal body temperature and normal external skin temperature. **Normal body temp. is 98.6 degrees F, and normal external skin temperature is 92 degrees F**

262.   What is the difference between protoplasm and proprioceptor? **Protoplasm is a jelly like substance within the cell and contains fat, carbohydrates, proteins and mineral salts; and proprioceptor is end organ of a sensory nerve fiber located in muscle and joints .**

263.   What can friction produce? **local hyperemia**

264.   TRUE OR FALSE. Flexion and extension can be performed as passive Range of Motion on the humeroulnar joint. **TRUE**

265.   Where is the olecranon process found?   **in the proximal ulna**

266.   What is a trigger point? **It is a hyper irritable spot that is painful when pressure is applied.**

267.   When you stimulate an active trigger point what can occur? What do latent trigger points do? **Active trigger points refer pain and tenderness to another part of the body, while latent trigger points exhibit pain when pressure is applied and don't refer pain.**

268.   Are neuromuscular lesions always hypersensitive to pressure? **YES**

269.   Neuro-physiological therapies utilize methods of assessing tissues and soft tissue manipulative techniques to do what? **To normalize the tissues and reprogram the neurological loop in order to reduce pain and improve function**

270.   If your client had arm abduction pain what would be affected? **The deltoid and biceps brachii**

271.   What are the two basic inhibitory reflexes produced during MET (muscle energy technique) manipulations?   **Reciprocal inhibition and isometric relaxation**

272.   TRUE OR FALSE. Isotonic contraction occurs with movement. **TRUE**

273.   What does SMB stand for? **Structural Muscular Balancing**

274.   Define what the following contractions are: Isometric, isotonic, concentric, eccentric. **Isometric muscle contraction is the contraction of a muscle in which shortening is prevented; muscle length remains the same. Isotonic muscle contraction is the muscle contraction in which tension developed in less than resistance of load, hence the muscle shortens. Concentric occurs when the muscle shortens during contraction.**

Eccentric occurs when the muscle lengthen during the contraction.
Note: There are two types of isotonic contraction: eccentric and concentric.

275. What are the three effects of hydrotherapy on the body? **mechanical, thermal and chemical**

276. What are the two categories of proprioceptors and where are each located? **Golgi tendon organs and spindle cells. The Golgi tendon organs are located in the tendon near its connection to the muscle and the spindle cells are located mainly in the belly**

277. What is a nerve plexus and where is it located? **A nerve plexus is a gathering of nerves and is located outside of the CNS (Central Nervous System.)**

278. When you flex the elbow, what becomes the antagonist? **The triceps**

279. Define muscle atrophy. **It is a degenerative process due to muscle disease.**

280. What is nephron? **The functional unit of the kidney.**

281. What are two responses to pain?   **Physical and psychological** Define mechanoreceptors. **Mechanoreceptors are receptors for vibration and for touch. They respond to mechanical stimulation or tissue distortion: touch, pressure, vibration, and stretch.**

283. Define organelle. **An organelle is a discrete structure within a cell, having specialized functions, a distinctive chemical composition and identifying molecular structures.**

284. What are mitochondria and what do they produce? **Mitochondria are the principal energy source of the cell, and contain the cytochrome enzymes for releasing energy and converting it to useful forms for cell operation. They produce adenosine 5'-triphosphate.**

285. What muscle initiates walking?   **Iliopsoas**

286. There are many muscle groups. What consists of the erector spinal group? **Longissimus, spinalis, and iliocostalis**

287. What muscles are involved in mastication? **Masseter, temporalis, medial pterygoid, lateral pterygoid**

288. Name the group of muscles of the shoulder? **Latissimus dorsi, teres minor, teres major, deltoid, supraspinatus, infraspinatus and the subscapularis**

289. What is the most superficial hamstring muscle? **The biceps femoris**

290. What is the difference between a sprain and a strain? **A sprain refers to damaged ligaments, and a strain refers to damaged muscles and tendons.**

291. Name the types of movable joints in the body. **Condyloid or ellipsoid, saddle, gliding, ball and socket, hinge, and pivot joints.**

292. Name three immovable joints in the body. **Suture, gomphosis, and synchondrosis**

293. What is synarthroses? **It is an immovable cartilaginous joint**

294. What does TMJ stand for? **It is a colloquial for Temporomandibular Joint Dysfunction**

295. What does TNTC stand for? **Too numerous to count.**

296. Name the divisions of the brain; the smaller & larger portions of the brain.
Celebrum, cerebellum, and the brain stem. The largest portion is the cerebrum and the smaller portion is the cerebellum.

297. What is inflammation and what are the four principal symptoms and signs of inflammation? **Inflammation is a protective and healing response that happens when tissue has been damaged. The 4 principal symptoms are heat, pain, redness and swelling.**

298. What are the three layers of connective tissue? **Epimysium, perimysium, and endomysium**

299. What is a subluxation? **An incomplete or partial dislocation**

300. There are several terms used describing body movement. Define the following. These are questions given on most any exam.
abduction = movement of a limb or body part further from or away from the midline of the body

adduction = movement of a limb or body part closer to or toward the midline of the body

extension = straightening of a joint or extremity so that the angle between contiguous (adjoining) bones is increased

flexion = bending of a joint or extremity so that the angle between contiguous bones is decreased

eversion = movement of turning a body part outward away from the midline

inversion = movement of turning a body part inward toward the midline

pronation = movement of turning a body to face downward or turning the hand so that the palm is facing downward

supination = movement of turning the body to face upward or turning the hand so that the palm faces upward

301. Name at least 5 positions of the body (positioning terminology).
Anatomic, supine, prone, lateral and oblique

302. What is acetylcholine?
A chemical neurotransmitter found at the myoneural junction

303. What are the names of the 3 abnormal curves of the spine?
Scoliosis, lordosis and kyphosis

304. Where is red bone marrow found and where is yellow bone marrow found? **Red marrow is found in the ends of the long bones and in flat bones i.e. skull and legs; and yellow marrow is found in the medullary cavity of the long bones**

305. There are two types of bone tissue, cancellous and dense. Where are both of these found?
Dense tissue is found on the outer portion of the bone just under the periosteum, and cancellous tissue is found on the interior of flat bones and in the ends of long bones.

306. What are the three most common types of arthritis?
Rheumatoid, osteoarthritis and gouty arthritis

307. Where is the mitral valve located? **Between the left atrium and left ventricle**

QUESTIONS ON THE CARDIOVASCULAR SYSTEM AND OTHER MISCELLANEOUS QUESTIONS

1.   What is carcinoma?
      The most common kind of cancer arises in the epithelium (the layers of cells covering the body's surface of lining internal organs and various glands.

2.   What is melanoma?
      An increasingly prevalent form of cancer which starts in the pigment cells located among the epithelial cells of the skin.

3.   Where do sarcomas originate?
      In the supporting (or connective) tissues of the body, such as bones, muscles and blood vessels.

4.   Where does leukemia begin?
      In the blood-forming tissues - the bone marrow, lymph nodes and spleen.

5.   Where are lymphomas born?
      In the cells of the lymph system.

6.   Would you massage a patient with cancer?
      Not before consulting with physicians who have knowledge of the case.

7.   Name the four components of blood.
      red/white blood cells, platelets, and blood plasma

8.   How many beats per minute is the (average) heart rate in an adult?
      75 to 80 per minute

9.   How many chambers are in the heart. **four**

10.   What is another name for "freckles"? **melanocytes**

11.   The conductivity of heart tissue is measured by what?
      an electrocardiogram (aka ECG)

12.   What does the cerebrum preside over? **will, reasoning, and memory**

13.   List 16 contraindications.
      high blood pressure
      low blood pressure
      varicose veins
      osteoporosis
      open sores
      diabetes
      any break or infection on the skin
      cancer
      burns
      inflammation
      fever
      asthma
      edema (in some cases)
      alcohol impairment
      extreme frailty and heart disease

LISTED ARE SOME OF THE NAMES YOU SHOULD BECOME FAMILIAR WITH AS EACH ONE IS IMPORTANT IN THE HISTORY OF MASSAGE

Dolores Krieger	Developed "The Therapeutic Touch" and (1976, April) Nursing research for a new age. Nursing Times
Jack Meagher	A physical therapist, and pioneer in the field of sports massage (pressure points) who also worked with animals on pressure points
Ruth Rice	A nurse, psychologist, and specialist in earl child development developed a specific stroking and massage technique for premature babies
Iona Marsaa Teeguarden	Researcher of acupressure techniques who developed Jin Shin Do
Pauline E. Sasaki	Teacher of advanced Shiatsu, co-author, translator and known world-wide for her work in Shiatsu
Hippocrates	Father of medicine, the Greek Physician
Bonnie Pruden	Myotherapy
Per Henrik Ling	Swedish massage, credit with developing it
Frances Tappan	Massage for physical therapy
Janet Travell	Trigger points, myofacial work
Milton Trager	Rocking motion, Trager Massage
Hwang Ti	Amma Massage
Albert Hoffa	Short massage in anatomical segments
Elizabeth Dicke	Connective Tissue Massage Therapy
James B. Mennell	Head of Massage Department @ St. Thomas Hospital, Londa 1934. Wrote a book on the basics of massage therapy
Ambroise Pare	Founder of modern massage
Sir William Bennett	In 1899he re-introduced massage to the medical profession and opened a massage department at St. George's Hospital in London
Murai and Mary Iino Burmeister	Jin shin jyutsu

NOTE: There are many individuals who have contributed to the massage profession. We suggest subscribing to the **Massage & Bodywork Magazine.** This magazine has the most current modalities, helpful articles and is an excellent magazine not only for professionals but for students who are preparing for their exams.

THESE TERMS RELATE TO PATHOLOGY
Acute "lower back pain"
Adhesions
Atherosclerosis
Arteriosclerosis
AIDS - HIV
Asthma
Migraines
headaches
gastroenteritis
constipation
sinusitis
hernia
PMS - Pre-menstrual syndrome
rotator cuff teat
myocardial infarction

sciatica
kyphosis
plantar fascitis
MS - Multiple Sclerosis
Osgood-Schlatters
leukemia
cerebral palsy
parkinson's disease
spinal cord injury - Para, Quad
burns
polymyositis
hypertension
rheumatoid arthritis
cystic fibrosis
systemic lupus erythematosus
congestive heart failure
patellofemoral stress syndrome
hypertrophic scar

CPR Review

1.   These common actions can lead to choking.
        **Drinking alcohol before and during eating
        trying to swallow poorly chewed food
        walking, playing, running with objects in mouth**

2.   What is the Heimlich maneuver and please describe it in detail?
        **It is the abdominal thrust that is used when a person is
        choking. There is an upward push to the abdomen given to
        clear the airway of a person with a complete airway
        obstruction. You ask the person if they are choking and if they
        can not respond tell them that you are trained in first aid and
        offer to help. Stand behind the person. The person may be
        either sitting or standing. Wrap your arms around their waist.
        Make a fist with one hand. Place the thumb side of your fist
        against the middle of the person's abdomen, just above the
        navel and well below the lower tip of the breastbone. Grasp
        your fist with your other hand. Keeping your elbows out from
        the person, press your fist into the person's abdomen with a
        quick upward thrust. Be sure that your fist is directly on the
        middle of the midline of the person's abdomen when you press.
        Do not direct the thrusts to the right or to the left. Think of
        each thrust as a separate and distinct attempt to dislodge the
        object. Repeat the thrusts until the obstruction is cleared or
        until the person becomes unconscious.   I highly suggest you
        take the American Red Cross Community CPR First Aid Course
        and review their workbook thoroughly!**

3.   What is a heart attack?
It is when one or more of the blood vessels that supply blood to a portion of the heart become blocked. When this happens the blood can't get through to feed that part of the heart. When the flow of oxygen-carrying blood is cut off, the cells of this part of the heart begin to die.

4.   If the heart stops what is this called? **A cardiac arrest.**

5.   The first aid for a heart attack is to do what?
Recognize the signals of a heart attack, make the person sit or lie down in a comfortable position, and call the EMS system for help.

QUESTIONS ON HYDROTHERAPY, APPLICATIONS, ETC.

1.   Define hydrotherapy.   **Hydrotherapy is the application of water in any of its three forms (vapor, ice, water) to the body for therapeutic purposes.**

2.   What is the purpose of the Russian bath and what are some of the benefits?   **The purpose is for causing perspiration as it is a full body steam bath and the benefits are improved metabolism, relaxation and cleansing.**

3.   What is the average time or duration for a cold bath, sitz bath/shower?
Approximately three to five minutes

4.   What is cryotherapy?   **Application of ice for therapeutic purposes**

5.   What are three things cold applications do that are beneficial to the body?   **Stimulate nerve, increase activity of body cells, and improve circulation.**

6.   Why would you not endure long periods of cold applications?
Because they can produce depressing effects

7.   What is a contrast bath and what are some of the benefits of a contrast bath?   **A contrast bath is alternating the application of hot and cold baths to a certain part of the body, and they help to increase local circulation. The causes an alternating vasoconstriction and vasodilatation of the blood vessels in the area being worked on.**

8.   Describe what an application of heat would cause and what a local application of heat would cause.   **The application of heat causes an increase in pulse rate, circulation, and white blood cell count. The local application of heat causes relaxation of local musculature and slight analgesia, increased metabolism and leukocyte migration to the area where heat is being applied.**

9.   What is a slight analgesia? **It is a neurologic state in which painful stimuli are so moderated that, though still perceived, they are no longer painful.**

10.   Give two objectives of hydrotherapy baths. **Stimulation of bodily functions and external cleanliness; increases local circulation either immediately or later; vasoconstriction or vasodilation of blood vessels.**

11.   What are three benefits of having a cabinet bath treatment? **Cleansing procedure, induce perspiration and relaxation.**

12.   Name the three classifications of effects of hydrotherapy on the body. **Chemical, mechanical and thermal**

13.   Give some reasons why the application of ice is beneficial. **Reduces pain, causes vasoconstriction to limit swelling, acts as an analgesic to reduce pain and is generally beneficial on swollen, inflamed and painful areas.**

14.   You should NEVER give hot or cold applications when a person has the following:
        diabetes
        lung disease
        kidney infection
        infectious skin condition
        cardiac impairment
        extremely high or low blood pressure

15.   TRUE OR FALSE. Hot water applications improve the condition of the skin by promoting perspiration and by increasing the circulation of the blood to the surface of the skin. **True**

16.   What would the temperature of a warm bath be in F and in C degrees, and what would the temperature of a hot bath be in F and in C degrees?
        Warm bath is 95 to 100° F which= 35 to 37.7° C.
        Hot bath is 100° to 115° F, which = 37.7 to 43.3° C

17.   What are the three main benefits of a whirlpool bath? **Soothes the nerves, relaxes the muscles, and increases the blood circulation**

18.   The skin can safely tolerate _____°F of hot water and approximately _____°F of steam vapor.   Water at _____°F over a prolonged period of time would raise the body temperature to a very dangerous level.   Fill in the blanks in order.
        115 ; 140 ; 110

19.   Define a Swedish Shampoo. **It is a body bath that cleans the body using either a brush or bath mitten solution of mild soap and warm water and is then followed by rinsing and drying the body.**

20. Is it okay to leave a client alone for long periods of time while they are in a cabinet bath? **No, you should always be near your client during water treatments.**

21. When is a salt rub usually given? **After a cabinet bath or after a hot bath. It can even be given as a separate treatment.**

22. Hydrotherapy baths are controlled by three things. What are they? **Proper temperatures, pressure and duration of the treatments**
                    END OF HYDROTHERAPY QUESTIONS

23. What is another name for the pelvic girdle? **Bony pelvis**

24. If a person says they have had depression for a long time and they think getting this massage will cure them, what should you do? **You should suggest they seek counseling, see their physician and also suggest massage.**

25. What hormone stimulates the thyroid?   **TSH**

26. What do tendons do? **Attach skeletal muscle to bones**

27. What part of the body is yang? **Upper part**

28. What part of the body is yin? **Lower part**

29. Is testosterone a steroid hormone?   **YES**

30. What do you do if you are working on a client and he/she complains of pain where you are working?
    release the pressure until they tell you they are comfortable

31. What are the sense organs? **touch, taste, smell, sight and sound**

SECTION VI

1.   Are there times when you should elevate a limb during massage? **YES**

2.   Define egestion. **It is the process of discharging undigested foods as waste.**

3.   Where does the gall bladder meridian begin? **outside cover of eye**

4.   Where does the spleen meridian begin? **at each big toe**

5.   What needs to happen to get rid of spasms and cramps in the posterior hamstrings? **Precede massage of hamstrings with anterior contraction of the quads.**

6.   What Yin organ is paired with the stomach meridian? **Spleen**

7.   Which meridian starts in the outside corner of the eye, zigzags and exits at the 4th toe? **Gallbladder**

8.   What would you send a doctor who has referred a patient to you? **A progress report.**

9.   What does HARA mean? **A centering place**

10.   What organ is related to metal? **Lung/Large Intestine**

11.   What meridian is most commonly used for headache relief? **L14**

12.   Which meridian is typically used for insomnia? **The heart channel is used for insomnia**

13.   What do you need to do if you are going into business with someone else? **File a K1 Report to the IRS.**

14.   In Ayruvedic practices the following is true. **The body and mind can not be separated**

15.   Why does a massage therapist drape a client? **It ensures trust in client and respects client's need for modesty.**

16.   Why is the appearance of a massage therapist important? **to develop trust, confidence and cleanliness**

17.   In which layer of skin are the lymph and blood vessels? **Dermis**

18.   What movement helps the functioning of synovial secretion? **Friction**

19.   What part of the body is affected by thoracic outflow syndrome? **Arm and neck**

20.   What does pes anserine mean?

       Pain and tenderness on the inside of your knee, just about two inches below the joint, are two of the symptoms of pes anserine bursitis of the knee. The pes anserine bursa is a small lubricating sac located between the shinbone (tibia) and three tendons of the hamstrings muscle at the inside of the knee. Because the three tendons splay out on the front of the shinbone and look like the foot of a goose, pes anserine bursitis is also known as "goose foot" bursitis.

21.   What is the function of neurotransmitters? **Inhibition**

22.   Bones touching bones are referred to as what? **grades of molding is a term used sometimes when bones are touching bones.**

23.   What is another name for SOMA? **Cell body**

24.   What systems insure homeostasis? **Respiratory and circulatory**

25.   What does it mean to have NET income? **Money minus deductions**

26.   What oil type is least likely to stain sheets? **Water dispersable**

27.   Therapists avoid injury to themselves by doing what? **Distributing their weight evenly between forward and back foot.**

28.   What muscle is affected when toenails curve up into shoe? **Flextor digitorum longus**

29.   Where does the bladder meridian/channel start? **Inner canthus of eye**

30.   In Chinese medicine, what organ is affected by edema, impotence, loss of memory? **Kidney and the heart**

31.   In what case would a doctor advise a "comfort order"? **For the terminally ill**

32.   What joint is affected by inguinal pain?   **Hip**

33.   If giving massage as barter, how much income do you report?
       Be sure and ask your instructors about this question. A student who sent in this question did not know the answer. The choices:
       100%

34.   How would you position arm to massage serratus anterior?
       Horizontally abduct

35.   Describe how you position pregnant woman in 3rd trimester.
       Side-lying

36.   What condition results in degenerative muscle turning into fatty tissue?
       Muscular dystrophy

37.   Give the term for one cycle of normal inspiration and normal
       expiration? **Tidal volume**

38.   What is aponeurosis? **Fibrous or membranous sheet connecting a
       muscle and the part it moves.**

39.   Where does the kidney meridian/channel start? **Under the 5th toe
       and runs to the sole of the foot**

40.   Where does the pericardium channel/meridian start? **It originates
       from the chest and enters the pericardium, then descends
       through the diaphragm to the abdomen to communicate with
       the upper, middle and lower Burner.**

41.   Where does the gall-bladder channel/meridian start? **At the outer
       canthus of the eye**

42.   Where does the liver channel/meridian start? **On the big toe and
       runs upwards on the dorsum of the foot and medial malleolus,
       and then up the medial aspect of the leg.**

43.   From where does the Direction Vessel originate? **The uterus (or
       deep in the lower abdomen in men) and emerges at the
       perineum.**

44.   The yang organs transform, digest & excrete impure products of what?
       Food and Fluids

45.   *TRUE OR FALSE.* The stomach and spleen are two meridians that are
       correctely paired? **TRUE**

46.   *TRUE OR FALSE.* The insertion point of the levator scapulae is the
       superior angle of the scapula. **TRUE**
47.   *TRUE OR FALSE.* Dr. Janet Travell was the founder of trigger point
       therapy. **TRUE**

48.   The yin organs store the pure essences resulting from the process of
       transformation carried out by what? The Yang organs

49.   The 5 yin organs store vital substances i.e. what? Qi, blood, body fluids
       and essence

50.   Do the 6 yang organs transform and digest or store. **They transform
       and digest.**

51.   Yang transforms what? **Qi**